Praise for *The God of Endurance*

"Comfort, one could argue, is the crisis of our age. The widespread avoidance of hardship—both spiritual and physical—has cast a shadow over the Church, her people, and the world at large. But Jesus Christ was never comfortable. He embodied the greatest act of love in history by pouring Himself out on the Cross, fully and painfully, without holding back. In *The God of Endurance*, Dan and Chase join forces to call readers back to this gritty and essential path—the way of Christ, who never ceased striving until His final breath. With wisdom and grace, they guide readers through the essential disciplines of staying spiritually sharp and physically strong. This book offers a practical blueprint for cultivating health, an ordered life, and an enduring, joy-filled soul. If you're looking for a true reset—body, mind, and soul—this is your go-to manual. Highlight it, dog-ear it, commit it to memory—and start living it."

—*Kevin Wells,* Author, *The Hermit: The Priest Who Saved a Soul, a Marriage, and a Family* and *Coached by the Curé*

"Dan Burke and Chase Crouse have encapsulated many sound principles not just for exercise and nutrition but for living a fully Christian life—for living as men and women fully alive for the glory of God. Whether you're just starting out in the spiritual life or well along that path, this book will help all who seek to live for the God of endurance."

—*Fr. Mitchell Athanasius Brown,* Pastor, Sacred Heart Cathedral, Gallup, New Mexico

"*The God of Endurance* is a must-read primer for Catholics seeking to improve their health and well-being. Dan Burke and Chase Crouse offer an integrated perspective that sets their work apart from the typical health books that concentrate exclusively on physical wellness. This book provides inspiration, practical advice, and actionable strategies to help you embrace exercise and nutrition as part of your spiritual journey to ultimately gain self-mastery."

—*Karen Barbieri,* Founder, Pietra Fitness

"*The God of Endurance* is an inspiring guide to growing in holiness by building physical, spiritual, and emotional strength. Dan and Chase combine their own stories with practical advice and a transformative road map to help you move with intention, care for your body, and use your time well. It's a down-to-earth yet powerful invitation to live with purpose, discipline, and faith. You'll also come away with a deeper appreciation for the incredible connection between body and soul."

—**Deanne Miller,** Cofounder, SoulCore

THE GOD OF ENDURANCE

DAN BURKE AND CHASE CROUSE

THE GOD OF ENDURANCE

A Practical Guide for Incorporating Exercise
and Nutrition into your Spiritual Journey

SOPHIA INSTITUTE PRESS
Manchester, New Hampshire

Sophia Institute Press
Box 5284, Manchester, NH 03108
1-800-888-9344
www.SophiaInstitute.com

Sophia Institute Press® is a registered trademark of Sophia Institute.

paperback ISBN 979-8-88911-528-1

ebook ISBN 979-8-88911-529-8

Library of Congress Control Number: 2025936157

Second printing

CONTENTS

*To my wife, Viva, the woman who taught
me what it means to fully give of myself and
to love like Jesus. Thank you for your total
gift to our family. This book is for you.*

Chase

*To my wife, Stephanie, the most beautiful woman
(inside and out) that I have ever met and my most
enjoyable partner in this effort to give all to God.*

Dan

Foreword

I (Dan) have been active all my life, even with many and serious health challenges, and I have always been an outdoors guy. For a brief time, I made a living (a poor one) playing and then teaching tennis. I was even able in my late teens to dunk a basketball, despite being only 5'10" tall. Yet outside of brief rehab stints for damaged knees or physical therapy routines for surgical recovery or other health challenges, I have not been able to develop a regular exercise discipline.

However, I was forced to reexamine my lack of exercise regimen after an incident that occurred while I was hiking on a very beautiful and mostly flat trail in New Zealand. At the end of the easy, fifteen-minute hike, I attempted to take a shortcut to the car. The effort consisted of a brief walk about two yards up a small hill—the equivalent of about six or seven steps up a staircase. But for the first time in my life (outside of specific injuries), I was unable to will my legs to climb the tiny incline. I was shocked. Yes, I had just begun to recover from a nine-month health battle related to my lungs that had rendered me very inactive. Yet even when I was only relatively healthy, I had never in my life been unable to make my body do what I wanted. I realized at that moment what it felt like to be feeble, to be old, to be vulnerable. It really shook me. Even through all my many hospitalizations and recoveries, I had rarely felt feeble, and only for very short periods. I could always will my way through recovery and find my way back to strength. But this time was different. I became awake to what the future could hold if I didn't make significant changes in my life.

Shortly after returning home, I looked at my calendar and realized that Lent was on the horizon. I thought, "Well, no time better than now." I knew I needed to use this time of self-sacrifice to strengthen my long-neglected physical health. As I began to reflect about how I might develop this new and very necessary habit, one thing was very clear: I knew I couldn't do it alone.

To me, any exercise routine always seemed too boring or too time consuming, or I didn't trust myself to understand the most efficient way to succeed. And if I didn't understand it all well enough to have confidence that I was doing it right, that every ounce of effort would yield results, it wasn't worth it. So I knew that I needed the same sort of sound guidance and accountability that I always recommend to folks who are struggling to overcome habitual sin or acquire virtue. I needed someone who was smarter than I was with respect to how to establish an exercise routine that made sense for my state in life and my medical challenges. As you might have already guessed, my coauthor and the primary source of expertise in this book, Chase Crouse, a devout Catholic and the founder of Hypuro Fit, is the man the Lord led me to on this new journey.

Much time has passed since that day in New Zealand, and because of God's grace, coupled with sound advice and accountability, I have succeeded in keeping the exercise commitments I started that Lent. In a short period of what I would call moderate but daily and deliberate exercise, I have quadrupled my muscle strength, my lungs and heart are improving dramatically, and I am actually beginning to enjoy exercise. By God's mercy, and this cooperation with His desire for me to be a better steward of the body He has given me, I feel better than I have in years. I still feel my age, but my "fitness age" measurement is getting younger.

To be clear, my goal most certainly is not to live longer but to live *better*. To better honor God by taking care of the body He has given me. My deep desire in this effort is to be able to energetically serve God and those entrusted to me until the day I die. While I don't control whether or not I will be able to fulfill this desire, I am very aware that if I fail to be a good steward of my body, I am sinning against both God — failing to love others as He has called me to, to treat our bodies as the "temple" within which He dwells (see 1 Cor. 6:19–20) — and my neighbors, since if I refuse to nurture my body, I will not be able to love them as God has commanded me. My prayer and hope for this book, then, are that if you have not yet made this same decision to be a better steward of the body God entrusted to you, you might be inspired and led to all the resources you will need to succeed, and if you have already come to the same conclusions that I had, that you will find your resolve strengthened as you read and discover new tools to help you on your journey.

One quick note about our culture. The exercise and supplement industry is booming. It's a money-making machine fueled by vanity and self-sufficiency. You may even have seen prominent Catholics in recent years begin to tout exercise and weight-lifting as a method of ascesis, which is self-denial for the sake of self-giving. They are right to some extent: exercise can be good ascesis. Even so, we must be very careful about our motives. While the world is right that exercise is good for you, we don't live according to the values of the world, and our stewardship must be motivated by our love for God and for those He has placed in our care. So as we jump into this adventure, we must adopt a purely Christian mindset about it. If we do, we can count on the blessing of God and the fruits of an authentically Catholic ascesis and avoid falling into the trap of being motivated by sinful vanity or fear.

With that said, if you are ready to break the habitual and destructive sin of the neglect of your "temple of the Holy Spirit" and live better for the Lord and for those you love, I believe you have the right guide in your hands. The next step is to learn—to orient your mind to truth—and to act, to bring your will into subjection to the truth; and that truth is none other than God Himself. So now let us look to Chase's story and begin this journey together.

Dan Burke

THE GOD OF ENDURANCE

CHAPTER 1

The God of Endurance and the Call to Holiness

*May the God of endurance and encouragement grant
you to live in such harmony with one another, in accord
with Christ Jesus, that together you may with one voice
glorify the God and Father of our Lord Jesus Christ.*

—Romans 15:5–6

IT WAS THE summer of 2012, and I (Chase) found myself on the floor of my bedroom, weeping, desperate, and alone. I had done everything a man was supposed to do during his first year in college: get the prettiest girls, party as much as I could, and develop a passion for college sports. I was imitating the male template showcased to me while growing up in Texas by both society and my family.

I had done it. I had checked every box. So why was I so miserable?

This was the question that had haunted me ever since I had moved back in with my dad for the summer. I had fallen back into the same crowd that I had hung out with in high school, and we had simply transferred all of our college stupidity back to our hometown for the summer. But soon the monotony of summer started to kick in.

One day, I was pacing around my dad's house trying to find something to do other than scroll cable TV (which I had already tried for an hour to no success). I had even tried looking into the fridge for a slab of bacon simply to pacify my boredom. Suddenly, I caught a glimpse of a book with an eye-catching cover tucked away on my nightstand. As you can imagine, I wasn't much of a reader in those days, but my boredom, and the Holy Spirit, led me to read something that would open my eyes to new horizons. The book was called *Rediscover Catholicism* by Matthew Kelly, and it had been lent to me by the father of an old high school friend who I had gone to church with.

Growing up I had been raised nominally Catholic: I was sacramentalized, but I definitely was not evangelized. I was forced by my parents to attend youth group and get confirmed, but I was the stereotypical punk kid who didn't want to talk in small groups. But after my Confirmation my sophomore year, I made some friends at the church and even willingly went to retreats and Steubenville conferences. The big feelings I got at these events might have been the Holy Spirit, or they could have simply resulted from the fact that I am secretly really empathetic and mirror the emotions expressed around me. (This is not only why I tear up while watching cheesy Christian movies but also why I can't watch cringe comedies: they make me too uncomfortable!)

By the time I got more into youth group, however, I was also slipping into the party lifestyle. At first, I didn't realize the two lifestyles were contradictory, but it didn't take long to put two and two together. Yet by the time I became aware of the problem, I was already trapped in my sin: the same sins of lust, hedonism, gluttony, and pride that would rule my world through my first year of college.

Back to the summer of 2012, and there I was staring at this book. At this point, I believed in God, and I would have told someone I was Catholic if they asked, but I hadn't been to Mass willingly in a very long time. But for whatever reason, this book stood out to me as something I should read, so I did.

If you've read *Rediscover Catholicism*, you know it's an easy read, and I didn't find anything groundbreaking in it at first. It simply helped me kill time while I waited for something I wanted to watch to come on the television. But then I got to chapter six, which unveils the idea of becoming the best version of yourself.

It forced me to ask the question: What does it mean to be a saint?

Thinking back to my old youth group days, I figured it was like an automatic up or down thing that happened when you died. But then the Holy Spirit stepped in and put the scariest question I've ever thought into my mind.

If I died right now, where would I go?

My answer: I don't know.

Cue the weeping alone in my bedroom. This was the first time I ever really thought about the fact that I would die one day. That one day I would have to answer for all of the times I spit in the face of my Lord when I committed sin after sin that I knew was wrong, sins that broke His most Sacred Heart, that made Him sweat Blood in the garden, that put the nails into His feet and hands.

I prayed my first real prayer that night. It was simple. "Lord, I'm sorry."

After I composed myself, I didn't really know what to do, so I called up my friend whose dad let me borrow the book, and he met me at the local Whataburger at midnight, and we talked for a couple hours about everything. He challenged me to run to the confessional, which I was terrified to do, and told me he'd help me set up a time with our parish priest, Fr. Skip.

I had known Fr. Skip since my early teens. He dropped everything he had planned the next day and heard my long and painful confession. He gave me the biggest penance I'd ever been given (still unmatched to this day!), and asked me to start coming to daily Mass.

I was a new man. Yet I was surprised a week later when an old temptation resurfaced. What the heck!? I had gone to Confession and was even starting to go to daily Mass! I shouldn't have to deal with temptation, right? That's not fair!

If only it worked like that.

Providentially, that same week I was white-knuckling my way through the time of temptation, a couple more old youth group friends asked me if I wanted to do one of those old Beach Body DVD workouts called *Insanity*. It was a sixty-day program dedicated to nothing but making you a giant pool of sweat at the end of each workout. I was in decent shape at the time, but this thing was tough!

But this is when I started making the connection between faith and fitness. I began to realize that if I could mentally *force* my body to go through this brutal workout that it didn't want to do, then in those times of temptation, I could mentally *stop* my body from doing the thing it wanted to do.

I could conquer myself in order to better give of myself. This inspiration was clearly from the Holy Spirit. Like many young Catholic men, I learned this lesson later than I should have, but that summer, a seed was planted, though it took more years to develop and grow. Nevertheless, for the first time in my life, I started living the law of self-gift. I was striving to conquer myself in order to one day give fully of myself to either the Church or my future bride.

The Law of Self-Gift

Many of the existential crises people face in today's world are caused due to a lack of a guiding rule of life, a trustworthy compass that can point us all in the right direction. People everywhere are stumbling blindly through life in search of their "purpose," and they end up falling into whatever camp happens to give them the most warm, fuzzy feelings at that particular time. These feelings-based pseudo-solutions then lead them to put on a certain pair of corrupt lenses through which to see the world.

The temptation to turn to the world for answers to life's problems is easy enough to understand, but it can be spiritually deadly in application. If the lenses through which we look neglect to empower us to see the goodness and dignity of ourselves and others, they don't come from the Holy Spirit. They don't come from the God who called everything He made "good" (see Gen. 1).

I don't know about you, but I don't want to see the world through a lens contrived by fallible humanity. The world and the people in it are too good, even if broken, to be viewed in any way that demeans them or deprives them of their God-given dignity.

One of the best things about being Catholic is that we have sure knowledge that Jesus has given us His Church to turn to when it comes to matters of faith and morals. The Church gives us a beautiful lens through which to see the world in the pastoral constitution *Gaudium et Spes*:

> Indeed, the Lord Jesus, when He prayed to the
> Father, "that all may be one ... as we are one"

(John 17:21–22) opened up vistas closed to human reason, for He implied a certain likeness between the union of the divine Persons, and the unity of God's sons in truth and charity. This likeness reveals *that man, who is the only creature on earth which God willed for itself, cannot fully find himself except through a sincere gift of himself.*[1]

This is the hermeneutic (interpretive lens) that Pope St. John Paul the Great used to view the world, and Scripture, through his work that we now call the Theology of the Body. He referenced this idea before he was pope in his work *Love and Responsibility*: "The 'law of the gift' is inscribed, so to speak, in the very being of the person. The entire tradition of Christian thought, for which the Gospel is and always remains the source of inspiration, convinces us about that."[2] Moreover, this law of self-gift wasn't something that was invented by the Church in the 1960s. *Gaudium et Spes* cites Luke 17:33 as inspiration for this law: "Whoever seeks to preserve his life will lose it, but whoever loses his life will keep it."

So what does all of this have to do with being a Catholic who takes exercise, health, and nutrition seriously? What does it mean for someone striving to grow in his ability to endure and say with St. Paul, "we rejoice in our sufferings, knowing that suffering produces endurance, and endurance produces

---

[1]   Pope St. Paul VI, Pastoral Constitution on the Church in the Modern World *Gaudium et Spes* (December 7, 1965), no. 24; emphasis added.

[2]   Karol Wojtyła, *Love and Responsibility*, trans. Grzegorz Ignatik (Boston: Pauline Books and Media, 2013), 281.

character, and character produces hope, and hope does not put us to shame, because God's love has been poured into our hearts through the Holy Spirit who has been given to us" (Rom. 5:3–5)?

Answer: everything.

To back up this big claim, let's go back to our catechism class for a bit. What is the point of being Catholic? My five-year-old would say: "Jesus!" And even though it's not the exact answer I was looking for, it really gets to the heart of the matter. To be united with Christ in Heaven is why we are Catholic. "To live in Heaven is 'to be with Christ.' The elect live 'in Christ,' but they retain, or rather find, their true identity, their own name" (*Catechism of the Catholic Church* 1025).

We know Heaven is the goal, and that entails being "in Christ." But what does it mean to be "in Christ"? Is that all we need to do? And is this a one-time thing, or a lifelong commitment? Let's take this one question at a time.

First, what does it mean to be "in Christ"? Fortunately, for most of you reading this book, it began when you were a baby. "For as many of you as were baptized into Christ have put on Christ" (Gal. 3:27). Through the sacrament of Baptism, we have been made into true children of God by putting on the humanity of Jesus. We become His brothers and sisters through the Holy Spirit. "Through Baptism we are freed from sin and reborn as sons of God; we become members of Christ, are incorporated into the Church and made sharers in her mission" (*CCC* 1213).

The next logical question is: then what? Is this all that needs to be done for us to enter Heaven one day? There are a lot of books written on the topic of justification and salvation, so for the sake of brevity I'll say this: yes and no. Baptism makes us sons and daughters of God, but children can lose their inheritance; in this case, through mortal sin (see *CCC* 1861). God gives us grace freely and initially at Baptism in order for us to respond to Him with our complete "yes," our total self-gift, but the road to Heaven lies in how much of ourselves we truly give back to God throughout our lives. We must cooperate with the work He has initiated in us in order to make it to Heaven. This cooperation entails an infinite number of moment-by-moment decisions to say "no" to our sinful nature and "yes" to what it means to truly walk with Jesus as an authentic disciple.

From the moment of Baptism, the call of the Christian is to do one thing and one thing only: imitate Jesus. To do what He did perfectly, namely, to give of Himself totally and completely to the Father. We too must freely give of ourselves so that we find total freedom in Christ. But what is this freedom? Let us look again to Pope St. John Paul II:

> Here we mean freedom above all as *self-mastery* (self-dominion). Under this aspect, self-mastery is indispensable *in order for man to be able to "give himself,"* in order for him to become a gift, in order for him (referring to the words of the Council) to be able to "find himself fully" through "a sincere gift of self."[3]

[3] Pope St. John Paul II, *Man and Woman He Created Them: A Theology of the Body,* trans. Michael Waldstein (Boston: Pauline Books and Media, 2006), 186.

This self-gift is impossible on our own due to the Fall, but Baptism gives us the life of Christ through the Spirit, and the Holy Spirit forms and shapes us into an icon of the Icon of God, Jesus, through our constant cooperation. This process is called sanctification.

So how do fitness and nutrition come in to the idea of sanctification? Here we need to look at the realm of asceticism, purposeful self-denial for the sake of self-giving.

> The word *asceticism* comes from the Greek *askesis* which means practice, bodily exercise, and more especially, athletic training. The early Christians adopted it to signify the practice of the spiritual things, or spiritual exercises performed for the purpose of acquiring the habits of virtue.[4]

I point this out in order to show you that we are not inventing something new and novel when we claim that the proper stewardship of our bodies is an inherently Catholic pursuit. St. Paul even says, "But I discipline my body and keep it under control, lest after preaching to others I myself should be disqualified" (1 Cor. 9:27). Proper fitness and nutrition are all about self-mastery and self-denial — asceticism — so that we can better give of ourselves and grow in sanctification.

---

4   Thomas Campbell, "Asceticism," ed. Charles G. Herbermann et al., *The Catholic Encyclopedia: An International Work of Reference on the Constitution, Doctrine, Discipline, and History of the Catholic Church* (New York: The Encyclopedia Press; The Universal Knowledge Foundation, 1907–1913).

But let's not fall into the classic mental trap of most moderns today: that this self-mastery will happen quickly. It would be pretty convenient if sanctification happened overnight. A simple zap of grace and *poof* you're all shiny forever. But we know from Scripture, Tradition, and our own broken experience that that is not how it works. God takes the initial and biggest step toward us, we have a free response to His grace, and then He, like a sculptor, slowly chips away at us until we reach the end for which we were all made: Heaven. As St. Francis de Sales wrote:

> I saw a piece of sculpture once that an artist had worked at for ten years before it was completed; during all that time with chisel and burin he never stopped chipping away at everything that was in the way of exact proportions. No, there is no doubt about it, we cannot possibly arrive in a day where we aspire to be. We have to take this step today; tomorrow, another; and thus, step by step, achieve self-mastery, which is no small victory.[5]

This all leads us to what the Bible says is one of the most important qualities you must have as a Christian: endurance.

---

[5] Francis de Sales and Jane de Chantal, *Letters of Spiritual Direction*, trans. Péronne Marie Thibert, ed. John Farina (Mahwah, NJ: Paulist Press, 1988), 155–156.

Endurance: The Proof of Love

Growing up in Texas in the 1990s meant that I was thrust into sports whether I liked it or not. It was just what kids did. Fortunately, I was naturally athletic and enjoyed competition, even though I really didn't enjoy physical discomfort of any kind. My mom and dad both fostered this competitive streak and were constantly shuttling us around to different practices and games without complaint.

My dad always had ESPN on the TV or listened to sports radio in the car. I learned to admire the greats of the 90s and early 2000s such as Michael Jordan, Nolan Ryan, and Andre Agassi. These were the legends of myth spoken of in my household. They were superstars of unbelievable greatness (at least in the eyes of my dad and seven-year-old Chase).

But what made them so great? Was it their strength? Was it their hand-eye coordination? Was it their size or speed? I'm sure those all had something to do with it, but each of the athletes above had very different builds and skill sets.

The thing that made each of these stars so successful was their ability to persevere—to endure.

Yet as great as these athletes were, their type of endurance is a mile wide and an inch deep. If you want to see a completely other-worldly level of endurance, look to the saints of the Church.

When we look to the lives of the saints, we find story after story of heroic endurance. From St. Thérèse of Lisieux's patient endurance of her illness and inability to travel the world to evangelize, to Pope St. John Paul the Great's ability to endure his forty-four-year battle with Communism, to St. Mother Teresa's decades-long suffering of the perceived absence of the presence of God while she nevertheless constantly served the poor and impoverished of Calcutta, these saints show us the true meaning of godly, courageous, and, above all, patient endurance.

The ability to practice patient endurance (*hypomonē* in the original Greek) has always been important in the Christian life, even at the very beginning of the Church. St. Paul wrote to the faithful in Corinth, "If we are afflicted, it is for your comfort and salvation; and if we are comforted, it is for your comfort, which you experience when you patiently endure (*hypomonē*) the same sufferings that we suffer" (2 Cor. 1:6). St. John in the Book of Revelation likewise addressed the church of Philadelphia: "Because you have kept my word about patient endurance (*hypomonē*), I will keep you from the hour of trial that is coming on the whole world, to try those who dwell on the earth" (Rev. 3:10).

Our first pope, St. Peter, also urged his readers to "make every effort to supplement your faith with virtue, and virtue with knowledge, and knowledge with self-control, and self-control with steadfastness (*hypomonē*), and steadfastness with godliness, and godliness with brotherly affection, and brotherly affection with love" (2 Pet. 1:5–7). The author of the Letter to the Hebrews puts it very bluntly when he writes, "For you have *need* of endurance (*hypomonē*), so that when you have done the will of God you may receive what is promised" (Heb. 10:36, emphasis added). That's right; without the virtue of endurance, we can't receive the reward promised to us, salvation.

The early Church had this knowledge, and the early martyrs lived this reality to the end. Their ability to endure was rooted in the theological virtues of faith, hope, and love. They believed that Jesus was truly their Savior, they hoped for eternal union with Him, and they loved Him so much that they were willing to sacrifice everything in this life to prove their love. To be like St. Sebastian, full of arrows and pain, yet not break or renounce his faith—what a gift that would be!

Yet many Catholics have lost this rugged virtue, this ability to patiently endure suffering for the love of God. Even if they may do it in one aspect of their lives, they fail to do it in the entirety of their being. We've fallen into the trap of modern convenience, which makes us confuse "easier" with "better." But patient endurance means saying yes to trials and difficulties and no to ease and comfort. However, this ability to say no for the greater yes has been not only lost in the Western world, it has been mocked as useless and replaced with self-centered pseudo-values that, instead of leading us to Heaven, open wide the gates of Hell. These are opposing pseudo-values of comfort and being taken care of rather than freedom and duty.

The Church is not sheltered from this mindset. I think of all of the priests I see who fail to take care of their bodies, and the witness of their failure, which shouts at us in plain sight, is that Jesus may be important to them, but maybe not that important. On the other hand, I think of the lay people who might take care of their bodies but who fail to spend dedicated time with the Lord in prayer because they are simply "too busy." It is truly heartbreaking to think of how many Catholics in the pews are living lives of hedonistic sloth when it comes to their spiritual or physical lives. I don't mean these observations to be a personal judgment or condemnation. The point is: the path of the Spirit is life and peace, and I want to offer you a way to live the life of abundance that Jesus has promised to those who resist the enemy and the flesh and embrace the difficult and narrow way to God.

You might be reading this thinking, "Chase, come now, I'm very busy! I have kids, a job, meals to prepare, and sports to take the kids to." Or maybe you're a priest reading this thinking, "He is a lay person, he can't possibly understand the demands that my parish places on me."

To the first objection, I will say that I am a husband, and my wife and I have three kids, two of whom are in gymnastics, and the other is one year old. I work a full-time job and run a side company with my wife. Yet even with the demands of my schedule, I go to adoration and work out every day during the week. Dan could offer the same testimony. He has managed several organizations of global size and impact, and yet he has made time for hours of prayer every day. Now he has added at least an hour a day Monday through Saturday for exercise. Where there is a will, there is a way—especially if it is God's will.

To the second objection, I've trained and worked with hundreds of priests who have almost all started out by saying the same thing to me: "I don't have the time." Yet most of them have embraced the challenge, and all now work out consistently while also growing in their prayer lives.

The lifestyle that we are inviting you to live, the life that we believe Jesus invites us all to live, requires healthy boundaries and the ability to say no to a lot of good, but unnecessary, things.[6] It also requires that you endure not only physical discomfort but also the discomfort of saying no to activities that would hinder your ability to love and serve the Lord in and through your state in life.

Our God is the God of endurance (Rom. 15:5). He invites us to live radically different lives — lives defined by our crosses and our ability to patiently endure them. To "run with endurance (*hypomonē*) the race that is set before us" (Heb. 12:1).

We want you to be like Jesus! To give of yourself totally to the Father in and through the Spirit. We are called to give everything: body and soul. This ability to give of yourself, however, requires you to have possession of yourself, because you can't give what you don't have.

If you pray consistently yet can't endure the physical discomfort of regular exercise, that's something to grow in. If you work out consistently but can't carve out time for personal prayer each day, that is also disordered. If you pray and occasionally work out, yet can't ever say no to alcohol or fried foods, you need to invite the Holy Spirit to help you grow in the virtue of temperance.

The bar is high for us in our Christian faith. "You therefore must be perfect, as your heavenly Father is perfect" (Matt. 5:48). It's actually *impossibly* high. And that's kind of the point. You can't do it alone, and you were never meant to.

So before moving on to more of the practical parts of this book, we would encourage you to run to the sacrament of

---

6   Dan's recent book, *Finding Peace in the Storm*, reveals that it can be just as problematic to pursue "good things" that are not God's will as it is to sin.

Confession. Run to grace Himself. Pray for the gift of patient endurance that is rooted in the love of the Lord and your family. Pray for the ability to conquer yourself in order to better give of yourself.

The journey to self-mastery will take a lifetime, because it's the journey of sanctification. Don't give up. Endure to the end!

"By your endurance you will gain your lives" (Luke 21:19).

Questions for Reflection

1. What stood out to you the most from this chapter?

2. When did you come to intentionally follow Jesus? Was it a specific event or a gradual growth in awareness?

3. What ways is God calling you to give of yourself in your current state of life?

4. What prevents you from fully giving of yourself? (Illness, laziness, addictions, time?)

5. If you have failed to care for your body as God intends, have you taken this sin to Confession?

6. What specific area of your life do you feel called to intentionally work on right now? (Spiritual, physical, nutritional, or relational?)

Consider your daily routine. Prayerfully ask the Holy Spirit to help you identify anything you can trim or change in order to make space for prayer or exercise.

STEP 1: MOVE!

Something Is Better Than Nothing

THE FIRST THING you need to know about exercise is that the best exercise is the one you can and will do on a consistent basis. To say this in another way that is more specific: you need to pursue a healthier life in the way that best fits your state in life, your means, your strengths and weaknesses, or whatever other factors are relevant for you to develop healthy habits.

At the same time, it is important to avoid any demonic ploys that will try to keep you from making a basic commitment to progress. The evil one will try to discourage you and remind you of your past failures. Or he will repeat the lie that you have no time.

There are many ways the enemy seeks to lie or distract us from living the life of freedom and self-mastery that God calls us to. But don't listen to the enemy. Instead, prayerfully reflect on any barriers you may perceive to even the smallest positive steps forward. Take these false barriers (that feel real) and write them down; bring them into the light of God's grace. Once you have them in front of you, renounce them in Jesus' name. Then affirm the opposite truth in Jesus' name. Here's what it might look like: "In Jesus' name, I renounce the lie that I don't have time to fulfill God's will for my life. In Jesus' name, I embrace the truth that though I may not see the way forward, if I pursue His will in His power, He will show me the way."

In the following sections, we are going to break down our preferred exercise styles based on the current data available and tons of personal and professional experience training real people. While we hope that the information in this section helps you build an exercise program and understand the why behind it, it's all for nothing if you hate it and aren't going to do it. We want you to own what you have. If the only thing you feel like you "own" are your two feet, then go for a walk. We would much rather someone go on a walk every day for twenty to forty minutes while chatting with a friend or listening to a podcast because that's what he or she genuinely enjoys doing and can in fact do regularly, than someone lift a dumbbell maybe once a month and does nothing else the rest of the time because he or she hates resistance training. Any kind of movement is better than no movement, and daily walks can yield dramatic improvements for those who were previously living a sedentary lifestyle.

But the fact is that obesity, which is loosely defined as being dangerously overweight, is killing people,[7] and we know that regular exercise, paired with healthy nutrition, is often the best medicine we have to save their lives. This isn't some new groundbreaking research. We have documented studies looking at intentional exercise and physical activities since the Morris "Coronary Heart Disease and Physical Activity of Work" study done in 1953.[8] Yet the obesity crisis

---

[7] Allison, D. B., et al. "Annual Deaths Attributable to Obesity in the United States," *JAMA* 282, no. 16 (1999): 1530–1538, doi:10.1001/jama.282.16.1530.

[8] Morris, J. N., and M. D. Crawford, "Coronary Heart Disease and Physical Activity of Work: Evidence of a National Necropsy Survey," *British Medical Journal* 2 (1958): 1485–1496, doi:10.1136/bmj.2.5111.1485.

in America started between 1976 and 1980, almost thirty years later! And when you look at the numbers, it just gets scary. In 1980, an estimated 13.4 percent of people in the USA were considered obese.[9] In 2008, that number jumped to 34.3 percent,[10] and the number is currently sitting at around 36 percent, according to the Harvard School of Public Health.[11] These are people who are actually *dangerously* overweight.

We are not saying that people who struggle with their weight are somehow inferior or "bad" in any way. What I (Chase) am saying is that as both a fitness professional and a Catholic who loves my brothers and sisters, I am begging people to wake up to the serious health risks of obesity. To quote just one medical study published back in 2009:

> Obesity is a significant risk factor for and contributor to increased morbidity and mortality, most importantly from cardiovascular disease (CVD) and diabetes, but also from cancer and chronic diseases, including osteoarthritis, liver and kidney disease, sleep apnea, and depression. The prevalence of obesity has increased steadily over the past 5 decades, and obesity may have a significant impact on quality-adjusted life years. Obesity is also strongly associated with an increased risk of all-cause

---

[9] "Obesity," Harvard T. H. Chan School of Public Health, https://hsph.harvard.edu/news/obesity/.

[10] Ibid.

[11] Ibid.

mortality as well as cardiovascular and cancer mortality.[12]

The fact that you're reading this tells us that you already have some sense of the need to improve your health. But we want to take it a step further than a mere "need." We would propose it is your duty to be as physically healthy as your vocation allows you to be. We're not saying we want you to be the next "six-pack Joe or Jane." We simply want you to have enough mastery of your body to serve God the way you are meant to.

For most people, this not only means losing the excess body fat that causes higher inflammation, insulin resistance, and reduced life expectancy. It also means gaining the adequate muscle you need to function properly—especially as you age. Even if you are younger, if you don't prepare well for that over-forty period of rapid muscle decline, you will suffer for your lack of preparation.

We understand that starting an exercise routine can be very intimidating for those who have never succeeded in doing so. And we want to help you succeed this time around. Your first goal should be to move your body in some meaningful way at least three times a week. Go for a hike, kayak, swim, play tennis or pickleball, jump rope, or box a kangaroo (just kidding ... kind of). We don't really care what it is as long as it is intentional movement done three times a week, consistently, over the course of your life.

[12] Xavier Pi-Sunyer, "The Medical Risks of Obesity," *Postgraduate Medicine* 121, no. 6 (2009): 21–33, https://doi.org/10.3810/pgm.2009.11.2074.

Remember, our bodies are gifts from God that are meant to be taken care of. "Or do you not know that your body is a temple of the Holy Spirit within you, whom you have from God? You are not your own, for you were bought with a price. So glorify God in your body" (1 Cor. 6:19–20). This is the first "rule" of this section on exercise: Your body is a temple worthy to be taken care of, so move it at least three times a week.

Resistance Training Is King

The digital age we live in has some really amazing advantages. Never before has someone been able to look up any question and have instant access to millions of free resources. But people have also never been more bombarded with poor or misleading information from self-proclaimed "experts."

Everyone knows through both anecdotal and personal experience that there is a lot of garbage out there. Anyone can post anything online, and most people that do are trying to sell you something. This is especially true of the fitness industry. Influencers with awesome genetics, years of experience, and the time to work out one to three hours a day are constantly trying to convince their followers that if you just do X, Y, or Z (while buying their product), then you too shall have the chiseled body of your dreams.

A lot of the workouts you see on Instagram, TikTok, or YouTube are usually not there for their technical excellence but rather for entertainment or click bait. You don't need to be doing all of these crazy workouts that involve ranges of motion and levels of athleticism that most people simply don't have (think of all the intense calisthenic workouts you see where people are shirtless and jumping all over the place). These influencers say, "Try this on your next workout." Then you try it, you can't do it, you get down on yourself, and you don't try working out again until the next time you feel "inspired." This can't be the best way to approach exercise, can it? We know instinctively that the answer is no.

We don't want to blow smoke here and "guarantee" you X result if you do Y program. What we want to communicate to you is what I (Chase) know through personal experience, innumerable client testimonials, and the data that are available to us through peer-reviewed studies.

A brief note about these scientific studies: Because of the amount of money to be made in the fitness industry, new studies are surfacing at a very fast pace—probably weekly at this point. But the information I want to set before you here is not of the pop-pseudo-science often spouted by "authorities" with something to sell (either for clicks or cash). I've looked at peer-reviewed, scientific explorations regarding everything from which exercise causes the greatest particular muscle growth, to how much time we should spend in cardio or resistance training, to how much weight we should lift. These authentic studies stand in contrast to those of the "experts" who make claims based on a false argument from authority and who may vaguely reference studies but who are mostly working to get you to believe something because they have something to sell—even if it is just their name. So in order to accept someone's assertion in this field, we should require that they cite specific sources, and if we want to be especially sure, they should cite multiple studies by separate, independent sources. This is all a bit of work that Chase has made a profession of and I (Dan) have had to pursue to convince myself that all this hard work is actually worth it. At the end of this book, we will give you a few sources that we generally believe are trustworthy in this realm.

With all of that in mind, authentic studies are pointing to the fact that resistance training is the pinnacle of all exercise when it comes to maintaining a high quality of life as you age.[13] Resistance training has one main goal: to build muscle. And while the threat of obesity is a serious one, being under-muscled poses an even greater risk. Dr. Gabrielle Lyon, board-certified doctor of osteopathic medicine (DO) with a master's in human nutrition, asks in her book *Forever Strong*, "Which does more damage, losing muscle or gaining fat? The answer is losing muscle. A study of elderly men comparing obesity with sarcopenia (age-related muscle deterioration) found that compared with high fat mass, low muscle mass both increased risk of injury and had a greater negative impact on performance."[14]

We don't want you to have muscle mass for vain reasons. When we speak of muscle mass, we are not referring to any images of professional bodybuilders that likely come to mind. Instead, we are talking about the muscle mass necessary for you to be healthy, have an active life, have fun, avoid falls, and live better until the Lord calls you home. We want

---

[13] See Kieran F. Reid et al., "Comparative Effects of Light or Heavy Resistance Power Training for Improving Lower Extremity Power and Physical Performance in Mobility-Limited Older Adults," *The Journals of Gerontology: Series A, Biological Sciences and Medical Sciences* 70, no. 3 (2015): 374–380, doi:10.1093/gerona/glu156.

[14] Gabrielle Lyon, *Forever Strong* (Atria Books, 2023), 35.

you to have proper muscle mass because muscles will keep you healthy the longest and will empower you to serve God and His Church.

An analogy Dr. Lyon uses is to think of your muscles as suitcases.[15] Within these suitcases, your body stores amino acids, carbohydrates, and fats. However, when there are too many of any of these three macronutrients, the suitcase will start to overflow. In the case of carbs and fats, this excess will be stored as body fat. A huge metabolic advantage of having more muscle is to make your suitcases bigger—which means that what would have been excess for obesity now becomes fuel for health.

The bigger your suitcase, the more likely you are to maintain a healthy weight and body fat percentage as you age. But your muscles aren't something to be purchased and kept indefinitely. There are several studies revealing how quickly you can lose muscle mass after not using your muscles.[16] Sarcopenia, or the loss of muscle mass, dramatically increases after the age of forty without proper protein intake and resistance training. It has even been shown that some individuals can lose between 1 and 3 percent of their lean body mass each year after the age of thirty. Simply think of how quickly someone can lose weight and muscle after having to spend a short time on bedrest at the hospital and this information shouldn't be too surprising.

If you aren't yet convinced at why having more muscles, and thus a lower percentage of body fat, can and should be a

---

[15] Ibid., 23.

[16] See Ogasawara et al. (2011).

priority, here is a list of the benefits you will see once you focus on building muscle mass:

* Increased metabolic rate (ability to burn calories)

* Improved insulin sensitivity (to help prevent type 2 diabetes)

* Enhanced strength and endurance

* Improved joint health

* Improved bone density

* Better cardiovascular health

* Improved mental health (fight depression and anxiety)

* Increased longevity and better quality of life

* Improved balance and coordination

* Less pain and struggle to get around (a huge issue after age fifty)

Okay, so you know that you should do something to help your muscles develop, but how should you go about doing that? This is where resistance training comes in.

Resistance training is a type of exercise that involves using resistance to force muscles to contract in order to accomplish a movement through a specific range of motion. Or, in layman's terms, it's using things such as your body weight, dumbbells, barbells, bands, kettlebells, suspension straps, or machines to load your muscles as you go through a movement pattern.

Okay, so that covers what resistance training is, but how often should you do it? How long should each session be? How do you plan an effective workout? And when should you change what you are doing? Let's answer these questions one at a time.

To the first question, how often should you do resistance training, we would argue for at least two days a week, but studies have shown that even one day a week can result in muscle growth and maintenance.[17] I (Chase) am a big believer in a saying from a professional bodybuilding coach named Joe Bennett: "Do as little as possible to get the most results." If you can get the results you need from one or two days a week of resistance training, a third day of cardio, and proper diet, then great! Especially if this is something you can maintain for the long run.

A crazy workout regimen that has you excited and working out four to six days a week can be great and sustainable for some, but if that's not you, then that is okay. When it comes to how often you need resistance training, the critical component is ensuring that it follows a schedule that you can follow most weeks of the year.

Let's assume you decide to start showing up to the gym (or your home gym) two times a week. How long should you work out? Well, that is determined by how you are planning and building your workout. If you are someone who has never worked out before, or hasn't worked out in a long time, we

[17] DiFrancisco-Donoghue, J., et al., "Comparison of Once-Weekly and Twice-Weekly Strength Training in Older Adults," *British Journal of Sports Medicine* 41, no. 1 (2007): 19–22, doi:10.1136/bjsm.2006.029330.

would recommend a more full-body workout. All this means is that you are doing one exercise for your legs, one for your chest, one for your back, and another for your shoulders.

Here's an example. First, do a warm-up of each exercise with a lighter weight. A warm-up set(s) is your chance to "practice" the exercise before you ask serious strain of your muscle during a working set. Start with a light weight and do 8–12 reps of the movement at a slow and controlled pace.[18] Really try to mentally engage the muscle(s) you are targeting. Rest a minute or so, then grab a slightly heavier weight and repeat. Gradually pyramid up the weight, and slightly lower the reps, until you are within 90 percent of your working weight (or, if it's your first time, until the weight starts feeling challenging around the 5-rep mark). Then, try the following (note that each set below does not include your warm-up set):

* Machine leg press: 3 sets of 8–12 repetitions with 90-second breaks between each working set

* Machine chest press: 3 sets of 8–12 repetitions with 90-second breaks between each working set

* Machine row: 3 sets of 8–12 repetitions with 90-second breaks between each working set

* Machine shoulder press: 3 sets of 8–12 repetitions with 90-second breaks between each working set[19]

---

[18] A "rep," short for "repetition," is a single execution of an exercise. One pushup is one rep, and ten pushups are ten reps. A "set" is a collection of reps. (E.g., if your goal is to complete twenty pushups, you might break your workout up into two sets of ten reps.)

[19] All of these sets do not include any warm-up sets.

All in all, this should take you approximately thirty to forty minutes to complete, depending on your warm-up.

Even if you are working out twice a week, you can repeat this exact same routine the second day in the gym. Spend the first few weeks getting used to the movements, figuring out good weights for you to use, and learning proper technique. Once you feel like you really have the hang of the exercises, shift your focus to pushing yourself hard enough so that you can't get to the twelfth repetition without some serious effort.

Next, how do you plan an effective workout? When planning an effective workout routine for yourself, the first thing you need to figure out, which we did above, is how many days you can dedicate to working out. The next step is to ensure that all of your primary muscle groups are getting attention throughout the week (legs, chest, back, shoulders). The rest boils down to your specific goals and experience level in the gym.

Let's take a client I have been working with for a couple of years; we'll call him Brad. When Brad first started working with me, he was about sixty pounds overweight and knew he could dedicate three days a week to the gym. His wife also encouraged him to join her on her morning walks during the workweek. Brad had some experience in a gym setting back in college, but he hadn't been back since then.

I started Brad on a simple, full-body workout like the one outlined above, and he did the *same routine* for three months. During that time, I helped him nail down form, taught him how to log and track his workouts, and eventually got him to really push himself when it came to making each working set really tough while maintaining good technique.

After the first three months, we transitioned him into what is called a PPL split (Push, Pull, Lower). Because he was working out three days a week consistently and enjoyed the progress he was making, this was a great option for him. This weekly routine (split) consists of focusing one day on your "push" muscles (chest, shoulders, triceps), another day on your "pull" muscles (lats, upper back, rear delts, biceps), and the last day on your legs (glutes, quads, hamstrings, calves).

Here is an example of what this PPL split might look like:[20]

✠ Monday: Push Day
- dumbbell chest press
- machine chest fly
- overhead machine shoulder press
- cable lateral raises
- cable triceps pushdowns

✠ Wednesday: Pull Day
- wide grip lat pulldown
- dumbbell low row
- cable high row
- machine reverse fly
- dumbbell bicep curls

✠ Friday: Leg Day
- seated hamstring curl
- seated leg extensions

---

[20] For examples and demonstrations of what these exercises are and look like, please see our YouTube channel at Hypuro Fit (https://www.youtube.com/channel/UCCkPhPgV8wrMXF-EgulM6NA).

- squat pattern of some kind (barbell back squat or front squat, goblet squat, Smith machine back squat, bodyweight squat)
- leg press calf raise

When you first start any new exercise routine, don't overdo it! It is not wise to push yourself too hard right out of the gate, especially if it's been awhile since you maintained a consistent workout routine. This is particularly important for people over fifty who have not been active on a daily basis. When you are younger, you can push and recover well enough even if you overdo it. But when you get over age fifty or so (depending on the person), if you push too hard and injure yourself, it can take a long time to recover, and this can be very discouraging. Pay close attention to your body as you begin to exercise. Soreness is fine; pain is not.

As you begin your new exercise routine, you want to manage your intensity by ensuring that you stay at or below the range of three to four "reps in reserve" (RIR). That means purposely stopping yourself before the exercise becomes too challenging. If the rep range is eight to twelve, find a weight where once you hit twelve reps you think to yourself, "I was starting to feel it by the end, but I definitely could have done more." Make a note of the weight you used, and rest for at least ninety seconds. Do one or two more sets of the exact same exercise with the exact same weight, and then move on to the next exercise. You should not feel too fatigued after these exercises are done. In fact, if you walk out of the gym and are only a little sweaty and thinking, "That wasn't too bad, and I definitely could have done more," then you did it right!

Keep this same intensity level, with solid technique, for your first four to eight weeks. That doesn't mean you can't up the weight. If the weight you started with week one becomes too easy by week three or four, awesome! You've just proven to yourself that your muscles are growing.

After four to eight weeks of three or four RIR, start to up the intensity and get closer to one or two RIR. That means that the last one or two reps should be tough! You should not be moving the weight on the last rep at the same speed as the first rep (no matter how hard you try). If you aren't making some funny faces and breathing hard after a working set, then it wasn't hard enough.

This fluctuation of intensity helps ensure that you provide enough stimulus to your muscles to keep them adapting and growing. This effort might mean you do eight reps of twenty-five pounds and hit the one to two RIR the first week. Then the following week you keep the weight and effort the same, but you get to nine or ten reps.

Progress.

Then the following week you keep the weight and effort the same, again, and hit twelve reps. More progress.

If eight to twelve reps was your goal, and you hit twelve reps the week prior, that is your cue to then up the weight and keep the intensity level the same. So you might go up to thirty pounds for seven or eight reps. And the cycle repeats. Keep the weight and intensity the same, and each week try to match or beat what you did the week before with a full range of motion and proper form. Then up your weights once you've hit your goal.

This leads us to the last question of how often you should change what you are doing in the gym. If your goal is to do as little work as possible for maximal results, then don't change the exercises you are doing for three to six months at a time (this is a wise approach for those over fifty). If, however, your goal is to simply show up and not get bored, it's totally fine to mix things up every two to three months. It is not wise to do something different every time you go to the gym, because then you are always trying to dial in the best form and appropriate weight without the ability to objectively log and see progress with your exercises.

Cardio 101

Resistance training focuses on your quality of life, and cardio training is geared toward longevity. There are ample case studies showing that people with a strong cardiovascular system tend to live longer than those who neglect it. In fact, the single most telling measure of the likelihood of living healthy and for longer is something called your VO2 Max, the maximum rate of oxygen consumption attainable during physical exertion.[21] This metric indicates how efficient your body is at distributing oxygen to your brain, lungs, and all of your muscle systems. The higher this number, the longer and stronger you are likely to live. Of course, we know as Christians that the Lord decides when this life is over, and we are not saying that this God-ordained appointment with our final judgment can be changed. However, as we exercise and pay reasonable attention to matters of health, we can reasonably assume we will live better during the time He has given us.

---

[21] The name is derived from three abbreviations: "V" for volume, "O2" for oxygen, and "max" for maximum. It is usually normalized per kilogram of body mass.

The reason we put cardio *after* resistance training is because, while it is very important, if all you do is cardio and you neglect resistance training, significant muscle deterioration is still going to occur as you age, and you can and will suffer from numerous aging ailments as you lose, or never develop, your muscle mass. In fact, it is best, within reason, to develop significant muscle mass *and* cardiovascular strength well before you reach fifty years old. Those who do will still suffer some decline (this is inevitable!), but the earlier you start to be a good steward of your body, the better it will treat you as you age.

With that caveat in place, let's talk about cardio!

With resistance training, efficiency (wise stewardship of the time the Lord has given us) is important. When it comes to cardio, the primary concern is getting it done in whatever way you enjoy the most (or hate the least!). This can be walking, jogging, biking, hiking, swimming, mixed martial arts (MMA), Brazilian jiu-jitsu (BJJ), playing tennis, or literally any form of exercise that elevates your heart rate for more than thirty minutes at a time.

Personally—we both hate running.

For both of us, running was always a punishment during sports when we were young, so unfortunately our subconscious still views it in a negative light. The same is not true for my (Chase's) sister, who loves running because she can "zone out, think, and pray." Cool for her, but I think she's crazy.

My (Chase's) preferred method of cardio is family walks, hikes, or MMA a couple times a week. As for me (Dan), I prefer pickleball or walking with a heavyweight vest (often called "Rucking").

The takeaway here is that you don't have to run for cardio. If you have "bad" knees or legitimately don't like it, then don't do it! Some people can white-knuckle their way through something they don't like and do it consistently for years on end, but most can't. You'll do it for a few weeks, but it will be extremely easy to find the smallest excuse not to do it when it's not convenient.

We hope this is a comforting thought for you, especially if you've struggled with cardio because all you've ever tried are those neighborhood jogs that you never really enjoyed. And if you're skeptical, just know that your heart doesn't know the difference between a jog and a hike, swim, tennis match, or kayak outing. It simply responds to the fact that your muscles need more oxygen in order to perform whatever task you are asking of them, and it speeds up or slows down accordingly. So again, it doesn't really matter what type of cardio you do, as long as you show up each time and do it!

The next question is how long and how often you should do a cardio workout throughout the week. If we take our baseline that we mentioned earlier of needing to do three days of intentional movement a week, with our hope that you are lifting weights one or two days a week, then doing cardio at least one or two days a week is a good goal.

If you're a parent with a crazy work schedule, we would encourage you to make these cardio sessions family-oriented, such as going on rosary walks or hikes. This can be easier said than done during the middle of summer or winter, but it's totally doable!

Just remember: whatever you decide to do, keep it simple and enjoyable, and that way it will be *sustainable*.

1. What stood out to you the most from this chapter?

2. What is your favorite form of movement? Was there a certain sport you played in school that you haven't done for a long time, or a certain activity you used to love?

3. When you start working out consistently, where is your preferred place to do so? Home or gym? Why is this the case?

4. What things in your life are not necessary and are getting in the way of dedicating time to exercise? What unhealthy time-wasters, such as social media, can you eliminate in order to meet your new exercise goals?

Make a plan. Look at your schedule for the next few days and carve out three days to move. For now, don't focus too much on balancing resistance training and cardio (we'll form more of a plan for that in chapter 4). Today, simply make a plan to move!

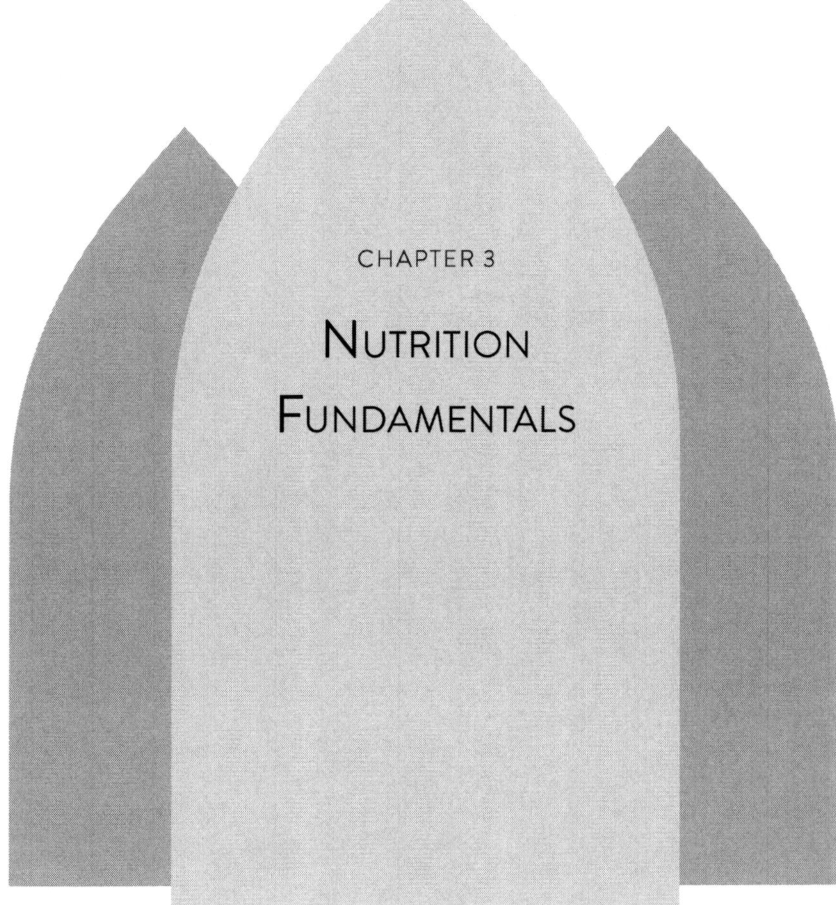
CHAPTER 3

NUTRITION
FUNDAMENTALS

IF EVER THERE was a topic that confused people about how to live a healthy life, nutrition is it. It can be so frustrating and overwhelming to try to sift through all of the different opinions and "studies" that people throw around these days on social media and even on news networks. It seems like at least once a month, Fox News or CNN brings in the newest health "expert" to try and convince you why this certain thing is bad and going to shorten your life and blah blah blah.

It gets real old, real fast.

What we want to do in this section is not dictate to you exactly how you must eat in order to be the next six-pack Joe or Jane. The first thing you need to understand about nutrition is that there is no cookie-cutter solution that works for everyone. Nutrition is more like a spectrum: on one side, you have foods that are nutrient dense, and on the other side, you have foods that are calorie dense.

You are not "evil" or "wrong" if you occasionally eat foods on the calorie-dense side of the spectrum. (Who doesn't love a good burger on a hot, summer day?) You are also not morally superior if you haven't eaten a French fry for the past two years because it was cooked in seed oil.

Nutrition is about choices. We are going to lay the groundwork for how to eat on the nutrient-dense side of things more often. But we also aren't going to tell you to never eat food you genuinely enjoy. Our goal here is to lay a foundation for you to implement, and understanding what you are willing to do when it comes to nutrition is a great first step.

Think about it this way: on average, most people eat three meals a day, making twenty-one meals in a week. If you can set up your schedule and eating routine so that nineteen of those twenty-one meals are nutrient dense, you are doing a great job!

Will this approach make you super shredded? Nope. Probably not. But will you be on the road to a healthy lifestyle? Yeah, you will be.

And we would also add that if you can't do the things in this first section consistently, then you really shouldn't be worrying about the more advanced, more nitpicky approaches to nutrition. The fundamentals must come first because these are the things you can and should do for the rest of your life, and how you approach nutrition at a root level needs to be sustainable and flexible. Yes, there will be times when it's okay to be more restrictive and disciplined, especially if you need to lose a certain amount of body fat in order to be in a healthy range. But assuming you hit that goal, or are already there, you simply don't need to be paranoid about every calorie for the rest of your life. Trust me, it gets old, and your in-laws will get annoyed.

Add before You Subtract

If you are reading this and have tried dieting over and over again with no long-term results, we would venture to guess that it's because you psych yourself up about starting a diet, get super excited about it, do it for a month or two, and then quit when life gets in the way. You go back to "normal" and then slowly but surely gain back whatever weight you had lost.

This can be exasperating, and we know instinctively that there must be a better way.

This brings us to our first rule when it comes to making a nutritional change: add before you subtract.

What are we adding? Protein. Lean protein to be specific. Foods such as steak, chicken breast, Greek yogurt, cottage cheese, protein shakes (*not* meal replacement shakes), pork, fish, eggs, shellfish, lamb, and wild game. Add it to every meal, because odds are, you aren't eating enough. There are also plant- and fish-based meal replacement options that provide high amounts of protein with minimal sugar. This is of particular interest as we go through seasons like Lent or regular fasts on Friday. We provide a list of these resources at the end of the book.

Protein is one of the three macronutrients that we consume on a daily basis. Two others are carbohydrates and fats. These macronutrients are the body's main sources of energy and the chief building blocks for your body to repair and grow its muscles, bones, organs, and nervous system. Micronutrients, on the other hand, include the vitamins and minerals that our body needs to function properly and optimally.

Recent estimates tell us that approximately 70 percent of Americans are protein deficient. We eat enough protein to survive, but not enough for optimal health. We simply think we don't need as much protein as we do. But remember, we want to live healthy longer. We shouldn't only eat what we perceive we need at this moment based on our desire or appetite. Instead, we should eat what we need with the long goal in mind — to build solid muscle mass both for the present *and* the future.

Protein helps us to develop lean body mass, manage our weight better, and improve our bone health. It boosts immune functionality, improves recovery, and supports healthy skin and nails. Another great thing about protein is that your body doesn't easily convert the amino acids that make up protein into fat. You either use it or excrete it. That's why you have bodybuilders eating 300 g (grams) of protein a day and keeping at 2 percent body fat. But the reason that "eat more lean protein" is the first rule of nutrition is because protein is the most satiating macronutrient. It makes you feel the most full.

Keep this fact about protein in mind before you begin any new diet or weight-loss plan. No one likes feeling hungry all the time. It's no fun. So if you can focus on getting 30–40 g of protein on your plate at every meal, you will not only feel full, but you will be more energized and be able to reap all the benefits protein has to offer, all while building muscle and losing fat.

So what does 30–40 g of protein look like at a meal? Here are some ideas:

* Breakfast: approximately 650 calories
  * four eggs plus one serving of egg whites = 30 g of protein (cooked with one serving of olive oil, which is only about the size of your thumb)
  * one or two turkey sausage patties = 10 g of protein
  * blueberries
  * whole wheat toast

* Mid-morning snack: 110 calories
  * protein shake: 20–30 g of protein

* Lunch: approximately 550 calories
  * Greek yogurt = 15 g of protein

- sandwich with five to eight slices of deli turkey or chicken on whole wheat bread = 15–20 g of protein
- Some easy veggies like carrots or cucumbers to go with it.

✣ Dinner: approximately 650 calories
  - 6 oz salmon filet = 35–45 g of protein
  - white rice
  - veggies (steamed or roasted with olive oil)

Your first thought when reading these ideas might be that this is a lot of food! And while it's a large *volume* of food, each individual meal or snack is not very calorie dense in itself. Everything above comes out to about 2,000 calories total. To put that into perspective, a number one (Original Chicken Sandwich and medium waffle fry) with a soda from Chick-fil-A is over 1,000 calories. Now we know that it is the Lord's sandwich, but that one, relatively small meal is half of your total daily calories! But eating nutrient-dense foods in place of calorie-dense foods allows you to actually eat more throughout the day.

Starting a new phase of eating with the approach of adding before subtracting will dramatically increase your odds of sticking with whatever change or restriction you put into place because it will be the first diet of your life where you will actually feel full. And if you feel full, you will be in a better mood and more likely to stick with good nutrition long term. So while this one addition isn't going to solve all of your weight-loss problems, it will be something you can sustain for the rest of your life.

Buying Food That Looks Like Food

It's human nature to want to figure out puzzles — to examine something we don't understand and then unpack all of its secrets. We become miniature Indiana Joneses in our own worlds. And I (Chase) have met so many people who approach nutrition like it's a grand mystery waiting to be solved. But at the end of the day, this next foundational principle will answer most, but not all, of your food struggles.

Namely: *buy food that looks like food.*

Walk into any grocery store, and you will notice that everything in the aisles comes in little boxes, cans, or bags. While not all of this food is calorie dense, it is processed in some way, shape, or form, and many of these packaged foods have been drastically changed from their natural state and often have added sugar, salt, fat, preservatives, or flavors. These highly processed foods are typically designed to be highly palatable. That means they are *designed to make you want to eat a lot of them.* And this is at the heart of the obesity crisis in our culture. Think of the last time you sat down and destroyed a bag of Cheetos and *still* felt hungry! These high-calorie processed foods aren't meant to make you feel full, which is why you tend to overeat them. To say this another way, you are being deliberately manipulated so that these companies can make money. And they are motivated to keep you fat and unhealthy.

But why should we capitulate to this evil when it not only causes profound discomfort (after we eat the junk) but also renders us unable to serve the Lord and others in our obesity and sickness?

Now not everything that comes in boxes or bags is "bad" for you. In fact, some good foods are actually "processed." And like we mentioned earlier, no food is inherently "bad" or "good." But there is a spectrum that you need to understand.

On one side of the spectrum, we have calorie-dense and, typically, *highly* processed foods. These include chips, sodas, candies, fried meats, cereals, most fast-food items, many desserts, and other super-yummy foods that we all know and love. If you're ever wondering whether a specific food falls into this category of highly processed foods, ask yourself a simple question: could I make or grow this on my own? If the answer is no, it's most likely a highly processed food we want to minimize. Think of an Oreo. You could make an Oreo-like cookie, but without the factory, there is no way you could replicate it exactly (especially because it's technically vegan!).

Once again, these foods aren't "bad," but they are *calorie dense*. That means you are getting a lot more calories per serving than you are of high-quality macro- or micronutrients that will feed your body and help it to be healthy.

We will never say that you should *never* eat these calorie-dense foods. There is a time and place. Think of days such as Christmas, Easter, birthday parties, and other celebrations. These are rare occasions when we want to celebrate. Even St. Francis of Assisi, when asked by his brother Franciscan priests whether they should abstain from meat on Fridays during Christmas, gave them leave to eat meat. It is actually disordered to fast on days on which the Lord calls us to celebrate. But once again, these are rare occasions. They are the exceptions, not the rule.

Now, on the other end of the spectrum, we have nutrient-dense foods: foods that have a lot of macro- or micronutrients and not a whole lot of calories per serving. This is where our rule for this section comes into play. Most foods that actually look like food at the grocery store are nutrient dense. These are fresh fruits and vegetables, lean meats, eggs, rice, steel cut oats, and basically any food that you see that is instantly recognizable as the food that it is. An exception here would be frozen fruits and veggies, as well as those canned in low sodium or zero added sugar. These are just as good and often more affordable.

At the end of the day, if the bulk of your meals can consist of fruits and vegetables, lean meat, and nutrient-dense carbs cooked in healthy fat sources (extra virgin olive oil is my go-to), you will be in a great place in your nutrition journey!

There was a client I (Chase) worked with in the past who was new to fitness and wanted to lose about thirty-five pounds. He had a little bit of experience in the gym but really hated cardio. Without blinking, I told him we could do this, and he wouldn't have to count one calorie, and we didn't have to do cardio if he didn't want to in order to lose the weight.

What was his first homework assignment? I had him make a mini food journal in which he took a picture of every-thing he ate beforehand and sent it to me. After a few days, the theme was clear: probably half of his food intake was ei-ther moderately or highly processed. So I had him slowly start replacing bags of frozen fried chicken with lean protein op-tions. He started adding fruits and vegetables in every meal. And finally, he replaced his more processed carbs such as chips, fries, and pastries with more nutrient-dense carbs such as rice, potatoes, corn, and steel-cut oats.

Sure enough, after only six months, my client had not only lost weight, he *gained* tons of muscle mass! He lost inches off his waist and was getting complimented left and right about how good he looked.

He was consistent with eating mostly food that looked like food when he bought it. He worked out three to four days a week. And I think the best part is, he still took his wife out on a date once a week to a restaurant where he ate yummy, calorie-dense foods with zero regrets.

If buying and cooking real, whole foods is a huge struggle for you right now, then you need to examine why. How are you prioritizing your time throughout the week? What can you say "no" to for the sake of saying "yes" to your health and wellness?

This approach might mean you say no to another episode of your favorite show, or you may need to plan out your week better than you currently are. It also might mean that you have to struggle through a few burned meals while you learn to cook.

Change is hard. And change can be viewed as "inconvenient." But this change, buying and eating mostly food that looks like food, is foundational to practicing temperance and moderation. You can't outwork the fork, especially for those of us whose high school metabolism has long gone bye-bye.

So how do you approach your week this way? Well, one of the easiest ways to go about planning your nutrient intake is planning around your protein source. Hopefully you have added protein at this point, so by planning around your protein intake, you can help alleviate a lot of the confusion about what to cook.

To practice, buy three or four lean protein sources for meals, such as chicken breast, lean ground beef (92% lean at least), salmon, and eggs or egg whites. Next, think of a few veggies that you like from a variety of colors, such as squash, carrots, tomatoes, red or green peppers, green beans, or brussels sprouts. Never force yourself to eat vegetables you hate. Find a few you like and stick with them.

Next step: pick three or four carb sources you want to use in your meals that week. Carbohydrates to buy are ones such as rice, quinoa, potatoes, sweet potatoes, fruits, and whole wheat (minimally processed) breads and pastas.

Finally, pick a healthy oil to cook with. Typically, you should use extra virgin olive oil for low-temperature cooking and avocado oil for high-temperature cooking.

Boom! You've got yourself a pretty solid grocery list.

If you aren't much of a chef, there are plenty of recipe sources and cookbooks out there. But just make sure the ones you use hit the above criteria about incorporating more lean protein and using food that looks like food, and don't forget to use salt (in moderation) and pepper!

These first two rules are so important that even if you just implement these and nothing else that we tell you, you will feel more energetic, lose weight, and perform better in your day-to-day activities. We guarantee it!

First Law of Thermodynamics and Understanding Weight Change

For many of us, weight loss is at the forefront of our thoughts when it comes to exercise and nutrition changes. That is literally the only way it has been marketed to people who have never actively tried to live a healthy, balanced life before. It feels like at least once or twice a week, the next health guru on social media tries to convince the audience why X food is evil and that "Program Y" is the "guaranteed fat loss program."

There are a lot of camps out there that guarantee fat loss by doing their programs. In the 1990s, it was the "all fats are evil" camp. In the early 2000s, it was the "carbs are evil" crew (this idea is still out there in the form of the carnivore diet). Most recently, we have the intermittent fasting camp, the keto diet craze, and the juice cleanse peeps. And here's the deal: If you have tried any of these diet plans, you probably have lost weight, at least in the short term.

The reason a person will lose weight with one of these diets isn't because of some metabolic "secret" or the fact that we need to eat like our ancestral caveman to be in ideal health.[22] The reason someone either gains or loses weight is because they were either in a calorie surplus or a calorie deficit.

This brings us to the first law of thermodynamics: energy cannot be created or destroyed, only transferred or changed.

Calories are simply how we measure the amount of energy we take in via the nutrition we consume. Our bodies

---

[22] Fun fact: there was a study done in 2011 that followed 229 hunter gatherer tribes and found that their overall dietary carbohydrate intake from sources like honey and wild berries ranged from 3–50 percent of their overall diet. A lot of this depended on what type of climate they lived in. So there is no one "caveman" diet, because each geographical and environmental region is vastly different in easily available resources. See Alexander Ströhle and Andreas Hahn, "Diets of Modern Hunter-Gatherers Vary Substantially in Their Carbohydrate Content Depending on Ecoenvironments: Results from an Ethnographic Analysis," *Nutrition Research* 31, no. 6 (2011): 429–435, doi:10.1016/j.nutres.2011.05.003.

burn calories just by being alive. It takes calories (aka energy) to breathe, sleep, eat, walk, type, read, talk—literally to do everything you do. This is why people sit around and aren't motivated to do much when they are malnourished: their bodies are trying to preserve as much energy as possible because they don't have enough.

If you have ever tried a diet before, this is also a reason why feeling motivated to work out is so tough after a while. Your body recognizes that it doesn't have enough energy via calorie consumption. It recognizes that if it moves at the same rate as before you started your diet, it will need to burn fat to maintain weight (which it doesn't want to do). So you will feel "less motivated" to work out because your body wants to stay in homeostasis. Coupled with concupiscence and related sins of the flesh, this can be a tough challenge to overcome.

Even so, if someone wants to lose weight, they *must* maintain a calorie deficit for an extended period of time. Being in a calorie deficit means you are consuming *less* energy than you are burning. And if someone wants to *gain* weight, usually to gain muscle mass, they need to consume *more* calories than they burn. To be clear, this is a scientific fact. Yes, it breaks most of what you hear out there about weight loss, especially all the excuses. Please allow us to say this in a way that we don't mean to be offensive or discouraging but is absolutely, incontrovertibly true: if you are overweight, it is because you consume more than you burn. There is absolutely no way around this fact.[23]

---

[23] We are not going to get into the weeds of various diseases or hormonal issues here. While these play an incredibly important role in weight management and health, it is beyond the scope of this book to dive too deeply into the topic.

Let's say that someone burns 2,000 calories a day without working out. That means that to lose weight, they would need to consume less than 2,000 calories a day for an extended period of time. How much less? Well, that depends on the person and how fast they want to lose weight while maintaining muscle mass.

Men can typically stand to be in a 250- to 500-calorie-per-day deficit and still function well. Women, due to hormonal health, typically should shoot for around a 200- to 300-calorie-per-day deficit. These numbers are a bit arbitrary, but they have to be because everyone has unique needs and goals. Even so, you need to start somewhere when it comes to tracking calories, and this is a good place to begin.

If someone is looking to add muscle mass, these numbers can be flipped. Adding 200 to 500 extra calories a day consistently, while consuming enough protein, and with adequate stimulus from consistent workouts, will lead to lean muscle mass growth. The thing you have to remember is to factor in the amount of active calories you burn while exercising.

For example, if someone burns 2,000 calories a day, then another 200 to 300 calories at the gym, that is a total of approximately 2,300 calories. In order to gain muscle, the person would need to consume 200 to 500 calories *more* than 2,300 calories.

If you want to learn how to calculate how many calories you burn, there are a million calculators online. Just look up "BMR calorie calculator" in any internet search engine, and you will find many helpful options.

At this point, you are probably asking yourself something along the lines of, "Do I need to count calories? What about counting 'macros' [macronutrients: protein, carbs, or fat]?" Well, counting macros is based on your overall calorie count. So if you want to count macros, then by necessity, you are counting calories.

You must be in a calorie deficit to lose weight, but that doesn't mean you have to count calories. Counting calories will take most of the guesswork out of your journey and will make things easier to calculate, but there are pros and cons. Here's a look at both:

* Pros:
  - The more accurate you are in counting and tracking your calories or macros, the more precise you can be with subtle changes in your diet.
  - If you start seeing results from counting calories or macros, you don't have to be constantly trying new things, because you know you are doing something right!
  - Counting gives you some wiggle room if you need to go out to eat for work or with family. If you know you have 700 calories left in a day, you can then find something with that many calories or less.

* Cons:
  - It is a bit tedious to do every day.
  - A lot of people tend to undertrack their calories (for example, they forget to calculate in the oil they cook with).
  - Some people become so overly fixated on tracking that it hurts them emotionally, mentally, or socially.

My (Chase's) business, Hypuro Fit, has had many clients who never track their calories and get amazing results simply because they stuck to our first two rules about protein and buying and eating food that looks like food. So if tracking isn't in the cards, and you've actually tried it for more than a week, then rest assured that you can still get some great results and be healthy without it.

At the end of the day, this is all to say that there is no magic diet that will reset your metabolism in order to "reach ketosis" and shed all fat from your body. It's calories in versus calories out—hard stop. Yes, hormones play an important role in weight management, because they influence caloric expenditure, but please don't buy something because someone on social media told you to. Always work with a health professional and an endocrinologist when making decisions about hormonal health.

We are not bashing any diets out there. A lot of people have gained energy and health by cutting out gluten, dairy, excess fats, processed foods, or whatever else a lot of fad diets have said you *have* to do. We simply want you to understand that the first law of thermodynamics is the reason for fat reduction or muscle growth.

Questions for Reflection

1. What stood out to you the most from this chapter?

2. What is your favorite food? Why is it your favorite?
   Is it nostalgic, do you associate it with something
   you enjoy, or something else?

3. How much protein do you think you eat on a daily
   basis? Make an educated guess, then try logging it
   for two or three days.

4. Why is it so hard for most people to stick with a
   diet? Why might the approach we outline above be a
   better option for most?

Make a game plan as outlined in the nutritional plan
above. Pick three or four lean protein sources for your
meals, then think of a few veggies that you like from a
variety of colors. Next, pick three or four carb sources you
want to use in your meals, and pick a healthy oil to cook
with. Based on these foods, come up with ten main meals
you can make this week (try to have a mix of breakfast,
lunch, and dinner options).

CHAPTER 4

PUTTING IT ALL TOGETHER

ONE OF MY (Chase's) biggest pet peeves with most self-help books is that they keep things in the theoretical and abstract. I understand why it's impossible to create tangible action items for everyone who might read a book. Authors would prefer to set up principles that can then be applied to the individual based on his or her best judgment, because that's really the only way to write a book for a lot of people. I get it, I really do.

But I don't want to end with an abstract chapter on nutrition fundamentals.

As I mentioned before, I want you to be the best version of yourself. I want you to live heroic virtue in the here and now. To be able to better give of yourself because you have started the road of self-mastery. I don't want you to start this path on Lent, New Year's Day, or a Monday. The best time would have been to start five, ten, or twenty-five years ago. The next best time to start is right now.

So this is where we're going to put together the principles we have outlined so far and give you a concrete game plan, a rule of life, for you to strive for self-mastery for self-gift. Will it be extreme for some? You betcha. Will it be hard for most? Yep. But will it be worth it? We guarantee it.

Sleep and Time Management

Shortly after my reversion to the faith, I (Chase) joined an organization called NET Ministries. We traveled the country putting on retreats for youth groups and Catholic schools. It was an extremely formative experience in a lot of ways, but mostly it was the first time in my life when I sought to serve a mission above and beyond my own selfish desires.

Before we were sent out, we spent about two months in training and spiritual formation. To be honest, I don't remember a lot of what we heard or discussed, but one line has always stuck with me: "A decision to stay up late is a decision not to pray in the morning."

No matter what your goals are, sleep is a critical element. From a muscle-building orientation, sleep is when the body heals and builds muscle based on the exercise stimulus that you gave it the day before. And when it comes to fat loss, sleep is the primary time when you lose fat.

Fat isn't primarily lost through exercise. In fact, exercise is a really inefficient way to "burn off fat." Even if you put yourself through a grueling hourlong workout and burned 500 to 700 calories, you can eat that with a couple of poor choices within minutes.

When you are in a calorie deficit, your body recognizes that you need more calories than you consumed, so it activates a process called lipolysis. During this process, your body will eventually oxidize fat in the mitochondria of your cells in order to tap into the ATP (a molecule that stores and releases energy) that is stored within the fat cells. The byproducts of oxidation are ATP (energy), water, and carbon dioxide. So if you are trying to lose body fat, sleep is critical, because you literally breathe out the carbon dioxide that results in fat burning when you sleep!

From a spiritual perspective, having a disciplined sleep schedule is vital in maintaining the proper start and ending of our days. We need to get enough sleep in order to be well rested and wake up ready to do God's will. St. Josemaria Escriva spoke of the importance of self-mastery in regard to sleep when he encouraged everyone to start the day with the "Hero's Minute," in which we do nothing but praise God for the first minute of our day:

> Conquer yourself each day from the very first moment, getting up on the dot, at a fixed time, without yielding a single minute to laziness. If, with God's help, you conquer yourself, you will be well ahead for the rest of the day.[24]

> The heroic minute. It is the time fixed for getting up. Without hesitation: a supernatural reflection and ... up! The heroic minute: here you have a mortification that strengthens your will and does no harm to your body.[25]

In order to have this heroic moment, you need to first go to bed and get enough sleep. How much sleep is the right amount? This will depend on the person's gender, age, activity level, and goals. The typical recommended range is six to nine hours. Women tend to need more sleep, while men can get away with not getting as much. Teenagers going through aggressive growth spurts will need more than their sixty-five-year-old grandfather who doesn't live a very active lifestyle.

[24] Josemaria Escriva, *The Way*, "Mortification," no. 191.
[25] Ibid., no. 206.

Our goal here isn't to dictate to you the exact number of hours you must sleep but to encourage you to practice *sleep discipline*. Beginning tonight, go to bed at a time that allows you to get from six to eight hours of sleep.

Sleep discipline means you have a "rule of life" in place that dictates the usual time you go to sleep and get up each day.[26] This rule will look different at various states of your life. If you are single or newly married without kids, you have the greatest control of your sleep discipline and should be stricter about it. For those parents out there whose babies and toddlers are unpredictable on the best of nights, your rule could very well be to simply get as much sleep as possible when it's possible.

I (Chase) encourage most of my clients to try to get their workout and prayer time done first thing in the morning, before work and family obligations wear you out and all you want to do after dinner is relax. This might require you to wake up earlier than you are accustomed to, which means you might need to adjust your bedtime to ensure you get the proper amount of sleep.

This is why we titled this section "Sleep and Time Management." The time management side of the equation is essential because we only have so many hours in the day.

---

[26] There are many practices that religious follow that laypeople can follow as well, and one of the most powerful is called a "rule of life." A rule of life is simply a commitment to God that we make, write down, follow, and examine on a daily basis in order to help us stay on track. Dan's book *Navigating the Interior Life* provides more detail on this powerful spiritual discipline.

You might be reading this and thinking, "This is nice in theory, but how can I possibly get up at 5 a.m. each day? That's way too early!" We would ask you to examine what time you are going to bed. Is it 11 p.m. or 12 a.m.? If so, then yeah, 5 a.m. would be pretty tough. So go to bed at 9 p.m. instead.

We can already hear the next thought: "Whoa! The kids go down at 8:30, and I need some 'me time' to recharge at the end of the day!" This is where I will give you an answer you probably won't like.

No, you don't.

You might think you need "me time," but you don't. You need to go to bed. Your family deserves a version of you that is well rested, physically active, and spiritually invigorated every day. Your family deserves the best version of yourself more than you deserve to watch Netflix or scroll on social media at night.

So when it comes to time management, we must set our priorities and non-negotiables. We won't presume to know what those are for you, but we can tell you what ours are:

✢ Chase's daily goals:

- Spend time in personal prayer; daily Mass as my schedule allows

- At least thirty minutes of intentional movement

- Two or more meals with my family (I work from home, so this is easier for me)

- At least thirty minutes of one-on-one time with my wife (usually right before bed)

- Seven-and-a-half hours of sleep (to bed around 9 p.m. and wake up at 4:45 a.m.)

- One to two hours of quality time with my kids (usually split up and sprinkled throughout the day)

✠ Dan's (empty nester) daily goals:

- Spend time in personal prayer; daily Mass most days

- At least one hour of intentional movement

- One meal with my wife

- Night prayer with my wife

- Seven hours of sleep (to bed around 8:30 p.m. and wake up at 3:45 a.m.)

As you can probably guess, we don't have a lot of time for extra-curricular activities. Yet even with these non-negotiables that I (Chase) have for myself, my wife and I make sure to give each other the breaks we need. She has a mom's book club she has been going to for years, and I get out once or twice a week to do MMA.

What are your non-negotiables? It's important to figure these out, because this will help you say no to the nonessentials such as Netflix and social media if needed for you to lead the kind of life that will make you fully alive.

Here are some categories to help you discern your non-negotiables (we would encourage you to have at least one or two from each category):

✠ How are you taking care of yourself spiritually?

- The Hero's Minute[27]

- Daily mental prayer

---

[27] The Hero's Minute is the first minute after your morning alarm clock. This is moment when you decide to get out of bed or hit that snooze button.

- Liturgy of the Hours
- Daily Mass / monthly Confession
- Spiritual reading
- Daily Rosary
- Nightly examination of conscience
- Spiritual direction

✠ How are you taking care of yourself physically?
  - Working out three to five times a week
  - Resistance training at least two times a week
  - Getting six to nine hours of sleep nightly
  - Daily walks
  - Getting seven thousand or more steps in a day
  - Cooking most of your meals at home with minimally processed foods
  - Drinking enough water (defined as drinking half your body weight in ounces of water a day)

✠ How are you taking care of yourself emotionally and socially?
  - Spending quality time with your spouse
  - Participating in parish life
  - Seeing a counselor
  - Participating in a small group
  - Organizing play dates with friends during which you can talk with other grown-ups while the kids play
  - Weekly date nights with your spouse
  - Chatting on the phone with a friend at least once a week

What can this look like? Here is my (Chase's) typical daily
schedule:

4:45 a.m.	Wake up
5:20 a.m.	Adoration (mental prayer and Liturgy of the Hours)
6:00 a.m.	Gym
7:30 a.m.	Breakfast with the family (my wife will go to the gym afterward)
8:00 a.m.	Play with kids or homeschool lesson with my oldest
8:30 a.m.	Morning offering as a family
9:00 a.m.	Workday starts
11:30 a.m.	Lunch with the family
12:00 p.m.	Angelus
5:00 p.m.	Dinner with the family
5:30 p.m.	Hang out with the kids
7:00 p.m.	Family Rosary (on some nights, this is when I leave for MMA or my wife leaves for book club)
7:15–8:00 p.m.	Bedtime routine with our three kids
8:00–9:00 p.m.	One-on-one time with my wife (watch something, read together, or play a board game)
9:00 p.m.	Bedtime

What I don't want you to do is simply copy and paste what I
do and assume this is the ultimate and most ideal schedule. It
is great for me and my family, but my situation isn't yours. I
give you a glimpse of what my life looks like in the hopes that
you can take the principles and ideas and apply them to your

situation. This will involve you saying no to a lot of things in order to give a greater yes to your family and vocation.

Yet another example of self-mastery for self-gift. Conquer yourself, and your schedule, in order to better give of yourself. To live the duty of the present moment to the best of your ability. To be a person fully alive and not a slave to your TV or cell phone, despairing over the fact that you have "no time" to take care of yourself physically, spiritually, and emotionally. You have the time—you just may not yet have the discipline to say no to the things that aren't as important.

Day 1: Going to Bed

While it's easy enough to say, "Go to bed!" most people, when they first try to go to bed earlier, will lay down and then stare at the ceiling and get annoyed at the fact that they aren't asleep after twenty minutes or so of trying. This is when a bedtime ritual comes in handy. These things won't magically solve all of your problems if you struggle with falling asleep. However, these practices, combined with the evening fatigue that comes from getting up earlier, will at least set you up for success.

The theme when it comes to a bedtime routine is actively doing things that bring calm and avoiding things that cause physical or mental stimulation.

Let's talk about the things to avoid first.

Let's assume the bedtime goal of 9:30 p.m. If this is the case, the biggest thing we want to avoid, starting around 8 or 8:30 p.m., is screens. The blue light from screens is extremely stimulating. That is why you can scroll and scroll on your phone and, before you know it, thirty minutes have passed.

This same stimulation is why toddlers are more prone to tantrums when they are in the middle of watching a show and you turn it off. It's almost like taking drugs away from an addict. The dopamine that they were feasting on is suddenly cut off, and they don't know what to do.

Put down the phone. Social media, the news, and work will all be there to welcome you with open arms in the morning.

The next thing to avoid is caffeine. Caffeine stays in the average person's system for four to six hours, and the effects of caffeine can even be seen eight or more hours after you drink it. Caffeine is most definitely a stimulant, and praise God for that after a night of wrestling a baby back to sleep. And while God was a genius when he thought up coffee beans, we shouldn't abuse them. If the goal is to de-stimulate, your last caffeine intake should be about six to eight hours or more before you hope to go to sleep. In the example of a 9:30 p.m. bedtime, that means no coffee after 3:30 p.m. at the latest. Ideally, I would recommend no caffeine after 1:00 p.m.

The last things to avoid are conversations, shows, or work tasks that involve a lot of brain or emotional investment, that is, are stimulating. If it's a weekend and you want to lose yourself in a philosophical conversation with a buddy over a whiskey, then go for it. But if the goal is to be in bed by 9:30 p.m. so you can wake up and get the day started right, then keep it simple.

You especially want to unplug and de-stimulate when it comes to anything related to work, something that you know will be waiting for you tomorrow. After 8 p.m., shut things down, make a note in your calendar if you need to, and then move on.

What can you do to actively de-stimulate?

This is a bit subjective, but we would recommend spiritual reading, or at least read a book, but not a thriller that is going to get your heart pounding. You can also set aside time for night prayer, the Rosary, reading your Bible, hanging out with your spouse, speaking to a loved one on the phone to catch up (only if this is something you find relaxing), taking a hot bath, drinking a cup of decaf or herbal tea or another hot beverage, or getting ready for bed.

You can also consider doing a Brain Dump. A Brain Dump is something I (Chase) learned from an author named David Allen in his book *Getting Things Done*. It is a brilliant technique if you, like myself, get stressed out when you are trying to remember and juggle too many things at the same time. I won't dive into all the details—buy his book for that—but here is how I do it:

Brain Dump:

1. Get a pen and paper (or use a notes app on your phone).

2. Set a timer for two minutes.

3. Once the timer begins, write down everything you can think of that you need to get done. This is *everything*: work, family, hobbies, friends, church, and so on.

4. Once the timer stops, put down your pen.

5. Look at your list of tasks. If there is anything on the list that takes less than two

minutes to complete (such as text a friend back), do it immediately.

6. Once all two-minute tasks have been completed, organize the rest of your list by location (emails happen at a computer, errands happen while out and about, conversations can happen at the office or at home).

7. Finally, organize your calendar to reflect when you plan on being at these locations and getting all of these things done.

This Brain Dump might not be the magic bullet for you, but for me it always helps me open a release valve when my brain gets too cluttered. Now that everything is out of my head, I feel set up for success to get to sleep in a timely manner.

So the first practical step we want you to take when implementing this book is this: *go to bed tonight at a time that empowers you to wake up early enough to pray and exercise.*

Month 1: Add Intentional Movement

Let's assume you set your alarm early enough to get in your prayer and workout. That's amazing! That is a huge first step, and even if you drag yourself out of bed the first week or so, I promise your body will eventually adjust to the new routine as long as you stick with it.

This first month, your goal is to consistently work out three days a week for at least thirty minutes at a time. As we discussed in chapter 2, it is ideal for you to exercise in the gym or with some form of resistance training. But if that is too intimidating for you right now, it's also totally fine to walk or hike to meet your thirty-minute goal.

The goal here is not to try to be "Shredded in Thirty Days," or to "Lose Your Tummy with This Thirty-Day Routine," or whatever other lies you see on the supermarket lifestyle magazine racks. The goal here is to lay a foundation, or form a habit, for something you can do for the rest of your life. We don't really care if you can do a thirty-day fitness blitz if that means you don't do anything again for a year.

Find an exercise routine that is sustainable, doesn't make you so sore you can't move the next day, and is hopefully something you even enjoy.

Here are three different routines, with exercises in them, that you can try to implement the first month:

1. *Walk and Body Weight Routine:*
    ◊ Monday: 30-minute morning walk (pray a Rosary or listen to a prayer meditation while you do it)
    ◊ Wednesday: bodyweight circuit and walk
       • Bodyweight circuit:[28]
          – Squats: 6–12 reps
          – Push-ups (these can be against a wall or on your knees to make it easier): 6–12 reps
          – Birddogs: 6 per side

[28] See Hypuro Fit YouTube channel or mobile app for demonstration videos.

         – 30- to 60-second break

         – Repeat for 10–15 minutes

     • Walk: 15–30 minutes

◊ Friday: 30-minute walk

2. *Walk and Home Dumbbell Routine*
   ◊ Monday: dumbbell full-body workout
   - Dumbbell goblet squat: 6–12 reps
   - Dumbbell chest press: 6–12 reps
   - Dumbbell low row: 6–12 reps per side
   - Dumbbell shoulder press: 6–12 reps
   - Rest 1–2 minutes between each exercise, and be sure to do some warmup sets before things get too tough
   - Repeat for 20–30 minutes
   ◊ Wednesday: 30-minute walk or jog
   ◊ Friday: dumbbell full-body workout (repeat the exact same routine you did on Monday)

3. *Gym Upper- and Lower-Body Program*
   ◊ Monday: upper-body day
   - Machine chest press: 3 sets of 6–12 reps with 2-minute rest between working sets
   - Cable lateral pull down: 3 sets of 6–12 reps with 2-minute rest between working sets
   - Machine shoulder press: 3 sets of 6–12 reps with 2-minute rest between working sets
   - Dumbbell lateral raises: 3 sets of 6–12 reps with 2-minute rest between working sets
   ◊ Wednesday: lower-body day

- Seated hamstring curls: 3 sets of 6–12 reps with 2-minute rest between working sets

- Leg extensions: 3 sets of 6–12 reps with 2-minute rest between working sets

- Squats: 3 sets of 6–12 reps with 2-minute rest between working sets (note: pick a type of squat you are comfortable with, such as dumbbell goblet squats, barbell back squats, Smith bar back squats, barbell front squats, leg press, or bodyweight squats)

- Leg press machine calf extensions: 3 sets of 6–12 reps with 2-minute rest between working sets

◊ Friday: Repeat upper-body day and begin alternating between these two workouts every time you go to the gym

This is your goal the first month: sleep and intentionally move three days a week. The specific days you choose don't really matter, as long as you are getting them in and are relatively consistent with them. Don't worry about cutting carbs, not eating sweets, or "dieting" yet. You simply don't have the mental bandwidth to program all of these new habits at the same time. That's why we have picked the most obvious ones first.

These workouts don't need to be the hardest thing you've ever done. You don't need to be drenched in sweat at the end of each one. You should not be so sore you can't move. If you are too sore, this is a sign that you pushed too hard out of the gate. By simply beginning to move in these ways, you will gain muscle and lose fat. We aren't trying to make you the next Arnold Schwarzenegger, we are trying to build a sustainable habit that you can maintain for the long haul.

Phase 2: Add Lean Protein

The reason this section is titled "Phase 2" and not "Month 2" is that it might take you more than a month to figure out a consistent exercise routine of three days a week *and* have it not feel like a huge burden. Both of those elements need to be in place for a habit to really start solidifying itself. If you are still dreading your activity, and it feels brutal trying to find the time for it, then you are still in Month 1 (or Phase 1). There is nothing wrong with it taking more than a month, so don't beat yourself up if it does.

When you have found a solid routine, it doesn't feel like a mental or scheduling burden, and you are starting to enjoy it (or at least not dread it), then this is when you have the mental bandwidth to add something else into your routine.

Namely: lean protein.

Here are your options when it comes to lean protein sources that we would recommend adding to your meals. You can have bigger servings than these, but these would be the minimums:

* 4 eggs (24 g of protein)

* 1.5 cups of egg whites (25 g of protein)

* 4 oz of lean ground beef (23 g of protein)

* 4 oz of salmon fillet (31 g of protein)

* 1.25 cups of shrimp (25 g of protein)

* half a chicken breast (25 g of protein)

* half a duck breast (29 g of protein)

- ✠ 4 oz of ground turkey (22 g of protein)

- ✠ 3 oz of NY strip steak (23 g of protein)

- ✠ 3.5 oz of lamb (20.8 g of protein)

- ✠ 4 oz of pork tenderloin (23 g of protein)

- ✠ 1 serving of no-sugar-added Greek yogurt (15 g of protein)

- ✠ 1 cup of cottage cheese (24.9 g of protein)

- ✠ turkey, chicken, or ham deli slices (1 serving is typically 9 g of protein)

- ✠ protein powder (only use if it has a minimum of 22 g of protein and no more than a few grams of added sugars and fats; do not use meal replacement shakes)

Foods people often associate with protein, such as nuts and beans, are mostly fats and carbs, and while these foods do have some protein in them, they should *not* be considered an appropriate protein source to add to your meals in this case. Eat them, but don't assume they are going to help your protein intake without also adding calories (and potentially adding weight).

Don't overly complicate this step of adding protein to your meals. For breakfast, drinking a smoothie with a scoop of protein powder is totally fine. Eggs with ground turkey sausage or cottage cheese with fruit is cool too. Find something you genuinely enjoy and have time for, and try out variations of that.

The easiest way to do lunches for my household is to purposely cook a lot of food at dinnertime and set aside leftovers to eat for lunch the next day or two. If this isn't possible for you due to having ravenous teenagers, or sharing a fridge with roommates, that is when you might need to meal prep or order from a macro-friendly meal delivery system.

Regardless of how you do it, the first step is simply to buy a variety of lean protein sources that you enjoy from the list above, then plan your meals around those protein sources. Don't worry too much about weighing out your protein to make sure it's exactly 4 oz or however much the serving size is. A trick I (Chase) learned from a company called Precision Nutrition is to use the palm of your hand as a measure of what approximately 20 g of protein is. Stick your hand out palm up, look at the circumference of your palm (not including your thumb and fingers), and that is about 20 g of protein usually (at least for an average-sized hand).

This isn't supposed to be rocket science or extremely precise. But if you can get one or two palms of protein on your plate at each meal, you're off to a great start.

Phase 3: Cut or Optimize

Now that you have the two foundational pieces in place, you have a decision to make based on your goals and where your health currently stands. The two options that you have before you are: to intentionally focus on cutting body fat, or to put your energy toward further optimizing your lifestyle or nutrition.

How do you decide which to choose? Let's do a bit of an examination of conscience here.

This examen will begin with a practical question: Are you medically overweight?

I'm not asking if you "think" you have fat to lose. This is not a subjective question. We are not trying to "fat shame" you into a weight-loss phase. We are asking you to objectively determine if, based on data, your body is holding onto more body fat than is medically healthy.

How do you figure this out? Let's start off with the simple numbers. Below are the generally accepted healthy body fat ranges:[29]

Age	20–29	30–39	40–49	50–59	60+
Female	16–24%	17–25%	19–28%	22–31%	22–33%
Male	7–17%	12–21%	14–23%	16–24%	17–25%

Now, figuring out if your numbers are above these ranges can be tricky. The most accurate way to figure out your body fat percentage is to get lab tested with a water scale or DEXA scan. However, most people don't have access to these, or they don't want to pay for them. The next best option is to work with your doctor at your next physical. Don't ask your doctor for your BMI (body mass index, which is calculated by dividing your weight in kilograms by your height in meters); this number is a total waste of time for most people. If BMI were an accurate sign of health, then almost every pro football player would be considered obese. Instead, ask your doctor

---

[29] This chart was pulled from Mayo Clinic.

for your body fat percentage using skin calipers or with a measuring tape using waist-to-hip or -height ratios. While these do not give you the most accurate measurement, they at least give you a starting point.

If you have a smart scale at home, be very careful about using it as a metric to determine your health. These scales use a slight electric pulse to measure your body fat percentage, but they often confuse water weight with body fat. So if you are going to use a smart scale, you need to weigh in first thing in the morning after you use the bathroom but before you eat or drink anything. And women should weigh themselves at the same point of their menstrual cycle every month to account for how the body holds onto water at various stages.

Okay, so we've answered the objective question of whether or not you are medically carrying too much body fat. Let's assume the answer is yes for the moment. Now the subjective question: Are you in a stable and good place mentally, emotionally, physically, and spiritually?

This means, are things in your life stable enough to enter into a season of intentional discomfort without it negatively affecting your mental health, your relationships, and your professional life? This might be something tough to figure out by yourself. Don't be afraid to speak with a counselor, spiritual director, spouse, or close friend to get another's view on the matter. Be okay with the answer being no. You already have the first two foundations in place: movement and protein. Which means you can still gain muscle and lose some body fat while getting stronger. You are already making progress!

If, however, the answer is yes, you are in an emotionally healthy and stable time in life to begin a cut, then buckle up! This is when real transformation (visually at least) begins to take place.

Here are my rules for an intentional fat-loss phase:

✠ The cut should only last 8 to 12 weeks. Then take a 1- to 2-week break from your diet, but NOT going back to just eating whatever you want. You should still be eating primarily whole foods and focusing on high protein, fruits, and veggies.

✠ Begin with Confession and pray specifically for the virtue of temperance and the Fruit of the Spirit of self-control.

✠ Protein and movement goals don't change.

- Shoot for .7 grams of protein per goal weight. For example, if my goal was to weigh 150 pounds, I would need to shoot for 105 g of protein a day.
- Intentional exercise 3 days a week. If that is all lifting, consider adding 1 or 2 days of cardio.

✠ No liquid calories.

- No alcohol, juices, milk, creamer, sodas, or sugary coffees.
- Exception: protein shakes are totally fine, as long as they aren't meal replacement shakes and have only a few grams of sugar or fat.

✠ No snacking between meals.

- No nuts, granola, peanut butter, cereal, chips, or whatever else you might snack on.
- Exceptions: you can "snack" on any lean source of protein, such as a shake, or on fruits and veggies with NOTHING added.

✠ No sweets.

- This one is probably obvious, but say bye-bye to cakes, candies, chocolate, donuts, and any pastry that is all sugar and no protein!

✠ Only eat out once a week, if at all.

- You are allowed one yummy meal a week (not a day). Make this something you genuinely enjoy. This is not only for the mental and emotional release valve that a yummy meal can bring. Having one day with slightly higher calorie intake can help with your metabolic health.
- Don't overthink what a yummy meal is, what is "allowed" or "not allowed." The only restriction I would give is to have no more than one alcoholic beverage at the yummy meal (if any at all).

✠ Focus on whole foods at your meals.

- Go back to our chapter on nutrition if you need to. You don't need to avoid all carbs and fats. Simply choose the ones that come from whole food sources at your main meals.

Now what if you answered "no" to either of the two questions above? What if you are not medically overweight or not in a stable place for a cut?

If you are not medically overweight but would still like to lose some body fat, the next question you must ask is why? Why do you want to lose the fat you have if your health is not in danger from it? Is it to look like a movie star? Is it to make you feel more wanted or loved? Is it to impress people you will never meet on social media? Truly confront yourself with this question of why before beginning an intentional cut when you don't medically need to.

Your answer might be that you simply want to challenge yourself and be as healthy as possible, which does mean a lower body-fat percentage. If that's you, then go for it. But this is our warning to you: there is a fine line between chasing optimal health for the sake of better serving your family and your vocation, and chasing a body composition for the sake of vanity. Be sure to have a good spiritual director to help you navigate your intentions here. You don't want your newfound path to health to become a doorway to sin.

Let's say that you don't have a need for a fat-loss goal, have discerned you don't need it for the sake of your spiritual health, or simply aren't in a place to take on an eight- to twelve-week cut. Here is what you can focus on instead: optimizing your health.

There are a lot of social media gurus out there pitching things such as supplements, eating raw liver, ice baths, saunas, and grounding. And while there might be some benefit to these, we are going to stick with the ones that have more authentic science to back them up and some direct experiential evidence from those whom I (Chase) have trained.

The list below is not intended to be exhaustive. But these are the aspects of life that are all important for us to focus on when we want to maintain a healthy lifestyle. What we recommend you do now is look through the list below and find three things that you would like to improve upon. It's okay if there are more than three that you *want* to work on at some point. But we only have so much mental bandwidth to form new habits, so only pick three for now.

- ✠ Recovery
  - Sleep discipline
  - Bedtime routine
  - Water intake/electrolytes (drinking half your body weight in ounces a day)
  - Stress management

- ✠ Faith
  - Daily mental prayer
  - Monthly Confession
  - More spiritual reading
  - Finding a good spiritual director[30]

- ✠ Nutrition
  - Eat mostly minimally processed, whole foods
  - Learn to cook (which will also require you to learn how to grocery shop!)

---

[30] SeekDirection.app is the best magisterium-faithful source for spiritual directors.

- Avoid alcohol and liquid calories
- Eat a wide variety of colors with fruits and veggies each day (eat the rainbow)
- Introduce supplements (creatine, vitamin D, fish oil, and magnesium are the only ones we recommend; exceptions for those with specific medical needs)

✠ Exercise
- Experiment with a variety of exercise splits (PPL, upper- and lower-body, full-body, "bro split," etc.[31]) to find one you enjoy the most and is most doable
- Work on sticking with a program for at least 8 to 12 weeks at a time to learn the art of efficient muscle growth and logging and tracking your workouts
- Introduce cardio once or twice a week if you aren't already doing it
- Introduce a recreational activity that you enjoy (soccer, tennis, hiking, pickleball, mixed martial arts [MMA], boxing, kayaking, etc.)

✠ Emotional/Relational
- Get plugged in to a good small group or community
- Make time weekly for a 1:1 date night with your spouse

---

[31] A "bro split" is doing one day per muscle group. For example: chest day, back day, leg day, shoulder day, and arm day. A PPL is a push day (chest, shoulders, triceps), pull day (back, rear delt, and bicep), leg day (glutes, quads, hamstrings, calves). An upper/lower split is alternating between an upper-body day and lower-body day.

- Take each of your kids on a monthly "date"
- Schedule a quarterly family weekend adventure
- See a counselor or psychologist
- Take time for yourself each day to recharge your batteries (hello, my fellow introverts!)

Let's walk through what this might look like for you. Say the three you picked were: water intake/electrolytes (drinking half your body weight in ounces a day), eating the rainbow of fruits and veggies each day, and making sure you have a weekly 1:1 date with your spouse. We can now break these down into the various skills and habits we will need to get them done.

Let's take drinking half your body weight in water each day as a test case.

The habit or skill we are trying to acquire is to stay consistently well hydrated. Do that by aiming for the goal of drinking half your body weight in ounces of water each day. Now let's break this down into practical tasks you will need to do in order to accomplish this goal and learn this new skill.

In his book *Atomic Habits*, James Clear describes what he calls "habit stacking." In short, if you want to learn a new habit, "stack" it on top of another habit you are already doing.

In the case of staying consistently well hydrated, habit stacking could look like this:

- Drink a full glass of water with electrolytes before you take your first sip of coffee (the coffee is the thing you are already drinking): 12 to 16 oz of water down.

✠ Drink a full glass of water at each meal throughout the day (you already eat): 36 to 48 oz of water down if you eat three meals a day.

✠ If you are already eating more protein and have started supplementing with a protein shake and are mixing it with water, we'll call that another 12 to 16 oz.

✠ Hopefully you have already started doing consistent intentional movement. I would always recommend drinking water right before, during, and after a workout. A normal water bottle has 17 oz of water.

The list above would get you to 77 to 97 oz of water a day. We could technically count any coffee and other liquids you drink, but for the sake of this exercise, we won't. If you are around 160 to 200 pounds or less, you have hit your goal! For taller, more muscular men, you might have to up the numbers above to hit your goal. And for those of you who are at the beginning of your weight-loss journey, remember that the goal of half your body weight in water is for lean body mass (or your goal weight), and not your total weight if you have more than 30 percent body fat. The same is true for total protein intake.

Regardless of which habits you want to implement to focus on optimizing your health physically, spiritually, or emotionally, follow the above practice of choosing your goal(s), breaking those goals down into habits and skills, and then breaking those habits and skills down into tangible tasks that you can stack on top of other tasks you are already doing. You're going to mess up (potentially a lot). Not every day will be perfect, nor does it have to be, and that's okay. But try again each day.

Lastly, we would encourage you at the end of each day to do a practical examen. This is essentially an evening examination of conscience with a focal point. If you are trying to stop doing something, examine your day and thank God for the times you avoided the temptation; or ask for mercy for when you failed to avoid it. If you are trying to add something, examine your day and thank God for all the times He empowered you to do the thing you are trying to do. The goal of this habit and prayer practice is to keep the thing you are trying to change at the forefront of your mind, and invite the Holy Spirit to give you the grace needed to change.

CHAPTER 5

CONCLUSION: THE BIG PICTURE

You might have reached this point waiting for our "big reveal." Our secret diet or workout plan that can guarantee success. Every other fitness guru and famous diet coach seems to have the system that will get you to the body of your dreams, so why don't we?

Because there is no secret system. No one is hiding anything from you. And if you see someone online telling you that they have the secret to guaranteed results—run away fast. No coach or trainer can guarantee you anything, because they aren't the ones who have to make the daily or hourly choices—that's you. Even if you saw a trainer in person three days a week for an hour each day, he or she would only be with you 1.7 percent of your week. The other 98.3 percent of your week would be on you to make the hard choices. To choose self-mastery for self-gift.

Our specific intention with this book is to help you to live a better life. We do not want to simply give you a few good ideas before you place this book on the shelf without actually implementing any of these changes. Simply knowing the things in this book won't actually make you a better person. As Pope Francis reminds us, "Thanks be to God, throughout the history of the church it has always been clear that a person's perfection is measured not by the information or knowledge they possess, but by the depth of their charity."[32] So hopefully by now you have decided to take your first step

---

[32] Pope Francis, apostolic exhortation *Gaudete et Exsultate* (March 19, 2018), no. 37.

forward, or to deepen your current commitment to exercise, holiness, and virtue and to become more of a gift of yourself to God and others. Either way, don't wait to start until next Monday or at some point in the future. Pope St. John Paul the Great said, "The future starts today, not tomorrow." So if you want to be a healthy person, start today. If you want to be better at prayer, start today. If you want to be a more loving spouse, start today.

The beginning doesn't have to be perfect. Don't let the perfect be the enemy of the good. It is not possible for a beginner to even be good at exercise, so don't set impossible goals for yourself and then allow the enemy to condemn you when you stumble or fall. And don't be afraid of beginning simply because you won't be good at first. The child isn't afraid of walking even though she isn't good at it. Instead, she lovingly and trustingly wraps her little hand around Dad's index finger and allows him to take some of the work of balancing and weight until she builds the strength and coordination to walk on her own.

So begin! Start! Go!

And once you have begun, keep showing up. If there is one secret that all the saints have shared in the history of humanity, it is that they show up—they endure until the end. Even when you feel like you have got the hang of prayer, exercise, protein, healthy eating, and whatever other habits you have chosen to work on, but then you fail, begin again. Be like St. Francis de Sales, who said, "Consider all the past as nothing, and say, like David: Now I begin to love my God." Yesterday counts for nothing. Today is what matters.

God has gone down on one knee and reached out His loving arm to you. He is proposing to you as a young man proposes to his future bride. He looks upon you as someone whom He loves more than anything, more than life itself. He has taken the first step; will you place your hand in His? Will you accept the universal call to holiness? Will you strive for self-mastery for self-gift?

The journey is a long one. But I hope that when we die, we are truly one with Christ in our heavenly home, and we can embrace each other in Heaven, knowing that we were given the grace to empty ourselves like Jesus did on the Cross. And through that grace, we truly found ourselves.

St. Paul calls our God the "God of endurance" for a reason. Growing in holiness takes time, effort, trials, and trust. We must patiently endure both our own shortcomings and failures, and those of others. If you try to implement everything in this book on your own, you will fail. Because we need grace. We need the Holy Spirit and the power only He provides.

We pray that the God of endurance gives you the graces needed to be a total and perfect gift of yourself to God and others. To give without counting the cost. To be like Jesus, His son, who showed us the way on the Cross. And with St. Paul we will say, "May the God of endurance and encouragement grant you to live in such harmony with one another, in accord with Christ Jesus, that together you may with one voice glorify the God and Father of our Lord Jesus Christ" (Rom. 15:5–6).

*"Indeed, the Lord Jesus, when He prayed to the
Father, 'that all may be one … as we are one'
(John 17:21–22) opened up vistas closed to human
reason, for He implied a certain likeness between
the union of the divine Persons, and the unity
of God's sons in truth and charity. This likeness
reveals that man, who is the only creature on
earth which God willed for itself, cannot fully find
himself except through a sincere gift of himself."*

Gaudium et Spes, no. 24

*"He calls each and every one to holiness; he asks each
and every one to love him: young and old, single and
married, healthy and sick, learned and unlearned,
no matter where they work, or where they are."*

St. Josemaria Escriva

1. What stood out to you the most from this chapter?

2. Whom do you need to talk to in order to hold you accountable to the game plan we described above? When will you talk to him or her? Don't delay, reach out today.

3. Do you have a spiritual director to speak to about your decisions regarding lifestyle decisions you want to implement? Do you know how to find one? (Check out our supplemental resources below for links to helpful resources.)

4. What time do you normally go to bed? Is that time conducive to you waking up in time to pray and exercise?

5. What do you do the last hour or two of your day? Are these things you need to do, or would your time and energy be better served doing something else?

6. What exercise plan are you going to implement? Do you have the resources needed to do this successfully?

7. Think back to the protein calculation you made at the end of chapter 3. Compare it to your need of 0.7 g of protein per pound of your goal weight. How are you doing? How can you improve?

Make a three- to six-month game plan as to how you are going to implement this book into your life. Share that with your accountability partner.

Afterword

It is important to note that when you start any spiritual discipline (which is how I [Dan] look at exercise), you are likely to experience some measure of consolation or encouragement in your new adventure. This was certainly the case for me. Even so, I also experienced desolation, both spiritual and physical. Desolation seeks to discourage us from doing what we have committed to do. And so I strongly encourage you, as you begin this new habit, to pick up and read or listen to the audio version of my book *Spiritual Warfare and the Discernment of Spirits.*[33] This book will help you understand the ups and downs of the consolation and desolation that emerge whenever we seek to orient ourselves more deeply to the will of God. The practice of discernment of spirits coupled with this new discipline will likely be a game-changer for you, because you will understand how to fight your desolation days to keep your commitments and how to ride your consolation days to victory. This practice is the simple but incredibly powerful pathway of the saints, the pathway of authentic discipleship, the pathway to honoring God with all that we are. May you know His presence and strength as you seek to give all you are to Him.

---

[33] You can also access a free video retreat at SpiritualDirection.com/Warfare.

I also unreservedly recommend Chase Crouse and Hypuro Fit to help you on your path to self-mastery. They are reasonably priced, faithful to a Catholic understanding of how we are to treat our bodies, and very helpful.

As you look for support in achieving your goals, keep in mind that you should seek out those who will help you develop healthy lives in both your body and your soul. These are just a few key factors that separate those who strive for self-mastery for self-gift from the rest of the pack:

1. They have a plan and commit that plan to God.

2. They examine themselves daily against that plan.

3. They show up no matter how they feel.

4. They never quit no matter what the setback.

5. They are accountable to another for wisdom, encouragement, and correction.

Resources to Help You Continue Your Journey

So that you can faithfully continue to study and fill your mind and heart with fuel for your new journey, we have assembled a set of resources that we have found to be helpful:

* Exercise, coaching, and insight:
  * Hypuro Fit (HypuroFit.org): Chase's Catholic fitness coaching.
  * Holy Habits app: This will help you establish a rule of life, track your progress, and be accountable.
  * Pietra Fitness (PietraFitness.com): Catholic stretching and exercise.
  * Soul Core (SoulCore.com): Rosary with stretch and strengthening exercises.
  * Hypertrophy Coach (YouTube.com/c/HypertrophyCoach): Bodybuilding insights.
  * Tom Purvis (TomPurvis.com): Exercise insights.
  * Wolf Coaching (YouTube.com/@WolfCoaching) (warning: occasional foul language): Sound, evidence-based resistance training.

* Spiritual growth:

- Holy Habits app
- *Navigating the Interior Life* by Dan Burke
- *The Fulfillment of All Desire* by Ralph Martin
- *Into the Deep: Finding Peace through Prayer* by Dan Burke
- *Into the Deep* film series (SpiritualDirection.com/Pray)
- *Spiritual Warfare and the Discernment of Spirits* by Dan Burke
- *Spiritual Warfare* film series (SpiritualDirection.com/Warfare)
- *I Believe in Love* by Fr. Jean D'Elbee
- *The Collected Works of St. John of the Cross* (Institute for Carmelite Studies)
- *Introduction to the Devout Life* by St. Francis de Sales
- The Avila Institute for Spiritual Formation (Avila-Institute.org)
- Apostoli Viae Community (ApostoliViae.org)
- To Find a Faithful Spiritual Director: SeekDirection.app
- To Find a Catholic Counselor: CatholicTherapists.com

✠ Nutrition:

- Hypuro Fit (HypuroFit.org)
- *Nutrivore* by Sarah Ballantyne (A book on a balanced eating approach)
- *Genius Foods* by Max Lugavere (A book on eating food for your mental health)

- *Forever Strong* by Dr. Gabrielle Lyons (A book on the importance of muscle and protein)
- *Gourmet Nutrition: The Cookbook for the Fit Food Lover* by John Berardi
- *Genius Kitchen: Over 100 Easy and Delicious Recipes to Make Your Brain Sharp, Body Strong, and Taste Buds Happy* (Genius Living Book 3)
- Dr. Layne Norton (biolayne.com)

✠ Lifestyle and time management:

- *Getting Things Done* by David Allen
- *Atomic Habits* by James Clear

✠ Supplement and food companies:

- Protein supplements:
  - TrueNutrition.com
  - OutworkNutrition.com
  - NoCow.com—Nondairy, plant-based
- Other supplements:
  - Creatine Monohydrate (for energy, muscle growth, and mental health)
  - Electrolytes (serviamindustries.com) (for hydration)
  - Vitamin D (healthy bones, immune support, and energy)
  - Magnesium (recovery, sleep, and energy levels)
- Food delivery companies:
  - Factor Meals (factor75.com)
  - Trifecta (trifectanutrition.com)

✠ John Paul II studies:

- *Man and Woman He Created Them* by Pope St. John Paul II
- *Love and Responsibility* by Karol Wjotyla
- *Witness to Hope* by George Weigel
- *The Glory of the Logos Made Flesh* by Michael Wolstein
- *Self-Gift: Essays on* Humane Vitae *and the Thought of John Paul II* by Janet Smith
- Theology of the Body Institute (tobinstitute.org)

About the Authors

Dan Burke is the founder and president of the Avila Institute for Spiritual Formation, which offers graduate and personal enrichment studies in spiritual theology to priests, deacons, religious, and laity in more than ninety countries and prepares men for the seminary in more than one hundred dioceses. Dan is the author or editor of more than fifteen books on authentic Catholic spirituality. To learn more, visit SpiritualDirection.com or ApostoliViae.org.

Chase Crouse's life took a pivotal turn in 2012 when he experienced a profound reversion to the Faith. Soon after, he joined NET Ministries as a missionary from 2012 to 2014, a period that sparked immense personal growth. Building on this foundation, he earned a bachelor's and a master's in biblical theology from John Paul the Great Catholic University. Following his studies, he and his wife moved to New York, where he discerned a calling to integrate Theology of the Body with fitness. As a husband and father of three, he understands firsthand the importance of nurturing both body and spirit. He is a Certified Personal Trainer (NASM), Functional Fitness Specialist (ACE), nutrition coach, and Change Psychology Specialist (PN1). Through his program, Hypuro Fit, he combines his spiritual, intellectual, and physical expertise to inspire others to embrace self-gift and personal growth.

Sophia Institute

Sophia Institute is a nonprofit institution that seeks to nurture the spiritual, moral, and cultural life of souls and to spread the gospel of Christ in conformity with the authentic teachings of the Roman Catholic Church.

Sophia Institute Press fulfills this mission by offering translations, reprints, and new publications that afford readers a rich source of the enduring wisdom of mankind.

Sophia Institute also operates the popular online resource CatholicExchange.com. *Catholic Exchange* provides world news from a Catholic perspective as well as daily devotionals and articles that will help readers to grow in holiness and live a life consistent with the teachings of the Church.

In 2013, Sophia Institute launched Sophia Institute for Teachers to renew and rebuild Catholic culture through service to Catholic education. With the goal of nurturing the spiritual, moral, and cultural life of souls, and an abiding respect for the role and work of teachers, we strive to provide materials and programs that are at once enlightening to the mind and ennobling to the heart; faithful and complete, as well as useful and practical.

Sophia Institute gratefully recognizes the Solidarity Association for preserving and encouraging the growth of our apostolate over the course of many years. Without their generous and timely support, this book would not be in your hands.

www.SophiaInstitute.com
www.CatholicExchange.com
www.SophiaTeachers.org

Sophia Institute Press is a registered trademark of Sophia Institute.
Sophia Institute is a tax-exempt institution as defined by the
Internal Revenue Code, Section 501(c)(3). Tax ID 22-2548708.